Drug
Regulatory
Affairs

Drug Regulatory Affairs

Gajendra Singh M Pharm, PhD

Professor and Dean
Faculty of Pharmaceutical Sciences
Pt BDS University of Health Sciences
Rohtak, Haryana

Gaurav Agarwal M Pharm, PhD

Head, Faculty of Pharmacy
RP Inderaprastha Institute of Technology
Karnal, Haryana

Vipul Gupta M Pharm

Technical Expert
Drug Regulatory Affairs

CBSPD

CBS Publishers & Distributors Pvt Ltd

New Delhi • Bengaluru • Chennai • Kochi • Kolkata • Lucknow • Mumbai
Hyderabad • Jharkhand • Nagpur • Patna • Pune • Uttrakhand

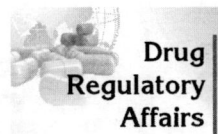

ISBN: 978-81-239-2881-4

Copyright © Authors and Publisher

First Edition: 2015
  Reprint: 2019, 2020, 2023, 2025

Published by Satish Kumar Jain and produced by Varun Jain for

CBS Publishers & Distributors Pvt Ltd
4819/XI Prahlad Street, 24 Ansari Road, Daryaganj, New Delhi 110 002, India
Ph: 011-23289259, 23266838   Website: www.cbspd.com
                                        e-mail: delhi@cbspd.com
Corporate Office: 204 FIE, Industrial Area, Patparganj, Delhi 110 092
Ph: 011-4934 4934   Fax: 011-4934 4935   e-mail: publishing@cbspd.com; publicity@cbspd.com

Branches

- **Bengaluru:** Seema House 2975, 17th Cross, K.R. Road, Banasankari 2nd Stage, Bengaluru 560 070, Karnataka, India
  Ph: +91-80-26771678/79   Fax: +91-80-26771680   e-mail: bangalore@cbspd.com
- **Chennai:** 18/8B, Subbarayan Street, Shenoy Nagar, Chennai 600 030, Tamil Nadu, India
  Ph: +91-44-42032115, 26681266   e-mail: chennai@cbspd.com
- **Kochi:** 42/1325, 1326, Power House Road, Opp KSEB, Power House, Ernakulam 682 018, Kerala, India
  Ph: +91-484-4059061-65   Fax: +91-484-4059065   e-mail: kochi@cbspd.com
- **Kolkata:** 147, Hind Ceramics Compound, 1st Floor, Nilgunj Road, Belghoria, Kolkata-700056, West Bengal, India
  Ph: 033-25633055, 033-25633056   e-mail: kolkata@cbspd.com
- **Lucknow:** Basement, Khushnuma Complex, 7-Meerabai Marg (Behind Jawahar Bhawan), Lucknow 226001, India
  Ph: 0522-4000032   e-mail: tiwari.lucknow@cbspd.com
- **Mumbai:** PWD Shed. Gala no. 25/26, Ramchandra Bhatt Marg, Next to JJ Hospital Gate no. 2 Opp. Union Bank of India Noorbaug
  Mumbai-400009, Maharashtra, India
  Ph: 022-66661880/89   e-mail: mumbai@cbspd.com

Representatives

• **Hyderabad**	0-9885175004	• **Jharkhand**	0-9811541605	• **Nagpur**	0-8692091830
• **Patna**	0-9334159340	• **Pune**	0-9664372571	• **Uttarakhand**	0-9716462459

Printed at Glorious Printers, Delhi, India

Contributors

Anshuman Agarwal
Faculty of Pharmacy
RPIIT Technical Campus,
Karnal, Haryana

Harshwardhan Khurana
Senior Research Analyst
Department of Strategic Regulatory
Services (SRS) United Health Group
Noida, Uttar Pradesh

Ish Grover
Assistant Professor
Faculty of Pharmacy
RPIIT Technical Campus,
Karnal, Haryana

Lakshyaveer Singh
Assistant Professor
Faculty of Pharmacy
MIP Rohilkhand University
Bareilly, Uttar Pradesh

Ms Shubhangi Bhilla
Product Executive
Product Management Team
Percos India Pvt Ltd., Delhi

Neeraj Kumar
Associate Professor
Devsthali Vidyapeeth College of Pharmacy
Rudrapur, Uttarakhand

PK Karar
Principal, Faculty of Pharmacy
RPIIT Technical Campus
Karnal, Haryana

Sandeep Kumar Singh
Assistant Professor
Department of Pharmaceutical
Science and Technology
Birla Institute of Technology
Ranchi, Jharkhand

Preface

This book is expected to be one of its kind to span a wide gamut of basics of pharmaceutics and drug regulatory affairs from the very traditional to what is the cutting edge technology today. This book is specially designed for graduate and postgraduate students of pharmacy. It contains a comprehensive description, an overview of existing knowledge of regulatory affairs and making it appropriate for industrial and institutional purposes.

Being an interdisciplinary subject, it covers a wide range of interests among the students, teaching community and pharmaceutical industry. Taking this increasing interest into account, the book gives a comprehensive introduction to the subject. The text not only deals with the basic concepts but also emphasizes technical and practical aspects.

The book contains numerous specimens, vivid illustrations, tables, diagrams and flow diagrams to present the concepts. The distinguishing feature is the glossary at the end of the book. In spite of great care, there might be some mistakes and deficiencies. We will be grateful for giving suggestions to improve upon ourselves. So kindly go through the content and do mail to us any observations at gbitsian@yahoo.com at your earliest.

Gajendra Singh
Gaurav Agarwal
Vipul Gupta

Acknowledgments

It is a moment of great pleasure and immense satisfaction for us to express deep gratitude and gratefulness to Dr Sukhbir Singh Sangwan, Founder Vice Chancellor, Pt BDS University of Health Sciences, Rohtak, for inspiring us to bring out this book.

We are especially thankful to Dr GN Singh, Drugs Controller General of India, for his all time support and encouragement.

We are indebted to Mr VK Arora, Ex-Vice President, Ranbaxy Laboratories Limited, Gurgaon, and Dr RS Jolly, Professor and Director's Grade Scientist, Institute of Microbial Technology (CSIR), Chandigarh, for their motivation.

Special thanks are due to our peers Dr SN Sharma, Dr SK Kulkarni and Dr Anupam Sharma for their moral support.

We express our gratefulness to Mr YN Arjuna, Senior VP (Publishing—Editorial and Publicity) and to Mr SK Jain, CMD, CBS Publishers & Distributors, for their sincere efforts in bringing out this title in time.

To our numerous students, whom we cannot possibly name individually, we greet them for their class interactions which have been the guiding spirit in selection of the subject matter and its logical arrangement.

Gajendra Singh
Gaurav Agarwal
Vipul Gupta

Acknowledgements

Contents

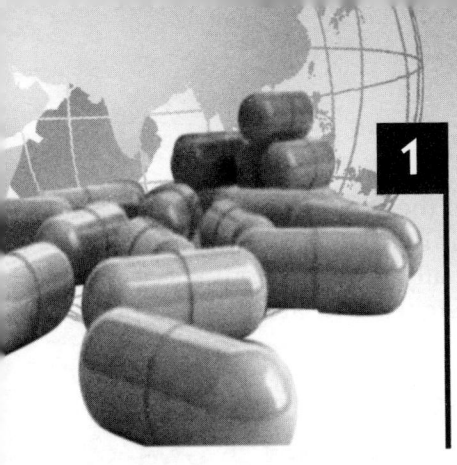

Introduction to Drug Regulatory Affairs

1

DRUG REGULATORY AFFAIRS

Drug approval process is a highly complex and lengthy process. In almost all countries of the world, packaged drugs may only be marketed with prior product-specific national approval. In this regard it is generally necessary to prove to the respective national regulatory authority the efficacy, safety and quality of a drug with extensive preparatory work and extensive documentation, also called dossiers. Drug regulatory affairs is a profession which protects the public health by controlling the safety and efficacy of products such as pharmaceuticals, biologicals, medical devices, veterinary medicines, over-the-counter (OTC) drugs, cosmetics and complementary medicines. The regulatory affairs departments of life-science companies ensure that their companies comply with all the regulations and laws concerning their business.

Regulatory affairs in the pharma industry may be defined as **"The interface between the pharmaceutical company and the regulatory agencies across the world"**.

OR

"The competent government agency which is responsible for ensuring that medicines work and are acceptably safe".

Although protection of public health appears to be a simple goal, but it is a highly complicated task and it can be achieved only through extensive and complex regulation. Safety, efficacy, purpose, risk/benefit and quality are the core principles which form an integral part of drug regulatory affairs. Drug regulatory affairs department is the backbone of pharmaceutical industry. Looking into the current scenario the regulatory affairs department has become one of the most important department for the pharmaceutical companies as it is the key interface between the company and the regulatory authorities.

Regulatory affairs department is involved in the development of new medicinal products, by applying regulatory principles and by preparing and submitting the relevant regulatory dossiers to health authorities. Regulatory professional obtains the marketing authorization for the product by presenting the registration document to regulatory agencies, and making the necessary subsequent negotiations. They contribute in the commercial and scientific success of the product development by giving strategic and technical advice, from the initial stages of the product development. Regulatory affairs contributes essentially to the overall success of drug development, both at early pre-marketing stages and at all times post-marketing (Fig. 1.1).

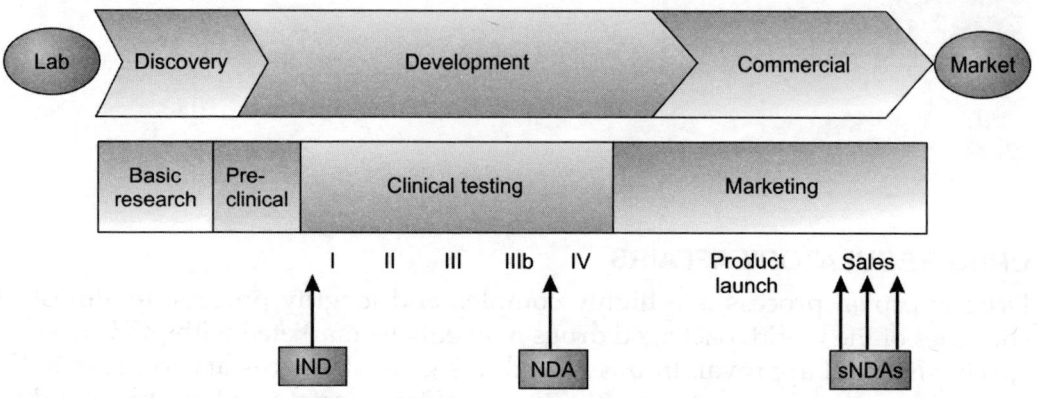

Fig. 1.1: Drug development process

The pharmaceutical industry deals with an increasing number of interesting drug candidates, all of which necessitate the involvement of the regulatory affairs' department. Regulatory affairs professionals can play a key role in guiding drug development strategy in an increasingly global environment. But, they also play an important operational role by considering the best processes to follow and enabling structured interaction with regulatory authorities. Consultations with the appropriate regulatory agencies, for example, scientific advice procedures in the European Union (EU) or pre-IND meetings with the food and drug administration (FDA), are milestones in product development. Regulatory professionals ensure that the information and data to be conveyed and discussed with the regulatory bodies are presented in the right way and form. They develop the regulatory strategy, arrange agency meetings, prepare and compile the questions and briefing documents; they attend the meetings and manage all communications with the agencies. Due to constantly increasing regulatory obligations and new requirements as well as the globalization of the pharmaceutical market, the demands and responsibilities of regulatory departments is becoming more and more complex. Today pharmaceutical companies are in a race to place new products on the market. The increasing costs of drug development are a major challenge for the pharmaceutical industry. Time to market is a critical index for pharmaceutical business and the key to return on investment. Acceleration strategies put tremendous pressure on regulatory departments since delays in approvals mean a massive loss in revenue generation. More than 15 years span is required to develop and launch a new pharmaceutical product in the market. During this scientific development many problems may arise. This process can be made fast by avoiding and solving the problems at appropriate steps only with the help of regulatory

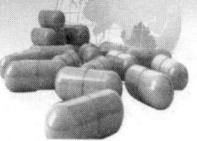

professionals. They help the company for keeping proper records, appropriate scientific thinking, update with changing regulatory guidelines/requirements and proper presentation of data.

Qualities of a Good Regulatory Affairs (RA) Professional

1. Commanding
2. Team player
3. Decisive
4. Practical
5. Good communication skill
6. Analytical skill—ability to evaluate the strengths and weaknesses of the technical and legal options open to a company.
7. Good informational technology skills
8. Ability to reapply scientific and regulatory principles
9. Ability to work with other disciplines
10. Flexible—always willing to learn.

Role of Regulatory Affairs Department

The below mentioned responsibilities are expected from a good regulatory affairs professional.

1. To keep up to the date record of company's product range.
2. To make sure that company's products comply with the current regulations.
3. To keep in touch with international legislation, guidelines and customer practices.
4. To keep track of the ever-changing legislation in all the regions in which the company wishes to distribute its products. They also advise on the legal and scientific restraints and requirements, and collect, collate, and evaluate the scientific data.
5. To prepare regulatory strategy for all appropriate regulatory submissions for domestic, international and/or contract projects.
6. To coordinate, prepare and review all appropriate documents, for example dossier and submit them to regulatory authorities within specified time.
7. To prepare and review of SOPs related to RA. Review of BMR, MFR, change control and other relevant documents.
8. To monitor the progress of all registration submissions.
9. To maintain approved applications and the record of registration fees paid against submission of DMFs and other documents.
10. To respond to queries as they arise, and ensure that registration/approvals are granted without delay. Impart training to R&D, pilot plant, ADI and RA.
11. To manage review audit reports and compliance, regulatory and customer inspections.
12. To help the company by keeping proper records, appropriate scientific thinking and good presentation of data.

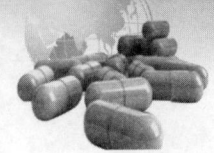

13. To provide physicians and other health care professionals with accurate and complete information about the quality, safety and effectiveness of the product.

Hence on the whole the Drug Regulatory Affairs department is essentially involved in the below mentioned activities (Fig. 1.2).

- Regulatory strategy
- Meetings with regulatory authorities
- Preparation, submission and maintenance of regulatory documents
  - IND, CTA, NDA, DMF
- Correspondence with regulatory authorities
  - Updates, safety reports, amendments, supplements
- Before clinical development
  - Preclinical phase
- During clinical development
  - IND
  - Interactions with regulatory agencies
  - Safety reporting
  - Updates
  - Preparing NDA
- Post-approval commitments
- During clinical trials
  - Filing of dossiers
  - Updates to data
    - CMC—product safety-related
    - Preclinical updates—new safety information
    - Clinical updates—adverse events/SAEs
    - IB, ICF, protocol modification
  - Meetings with regulators
    - Updates
    - Change in plans/strategy
    - Seeking advice
- After clinical trials—preparing for NDA
  - Dossiers—CTD format
    - Writing
    - Compilation
    - Publishing
    - Submission
  - Interaction with regulators during review
  - Label negotiation
  - Product launch
- After product launch
  - Product quality
    - Reporting changes as per guidelines

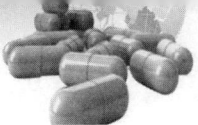

- Product safety
  - Pharmacovigilance

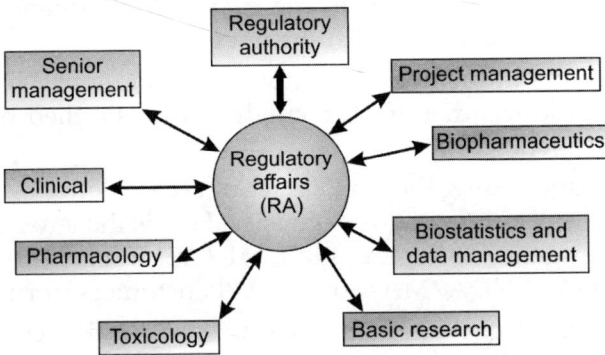

Fig 1.2: Role of RA in drug development

Types, formats and contents of submissions that RA department is being involved in:

- IND
- NDA
- ANDA
- DMF
- CTA
- Annual reports
- Compliance aspects—GXPs, that RA department is being involved in :
  - GLPs—good laboratory practices—need to be followed in the preclinical studies.
  - GMPs—good manufacturing practices—need to be followed in the clinical and market
  - GCP—good clinical practices—need to be followed in the clinical studies.

All the compliance aspects mentioned above are applicable throughout the drug developments and non-compliance will lead to serious consequences.

Job of a regulatory affairs professional in an API (active pharmaceutical ingredient) manufacturing company:

1. Filing a DMF/ASMF with regulatory agencies in support of the NDA/ANDA/INDA/MAA filed by a formulator (drug product manufacturer who uses API of that particular API manufacturing company).
2. Filing dossier of API with EDQM for obtaining CEP.
3. Assessing and filing amendments/variations to the information (which may be related to manufacture, control, stability studies, etc.) in DMF/ASMF/dossier of particular API with the regulatory agencies. Major amendments are to be reported prior to their implementation while minor amendments may be reported annually. The classification of amendments will be dealt in the later posts.

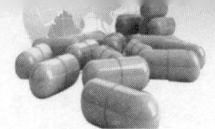

4. Taking approval of customers of API before implementing any major changes regarding the information mentioned in DMF/ASMF/dossier. The updated DMF/ASMF may be submitted to the customer simultaneously along with amendments/variations filed with the agency.

5. Preparing and submitting open part/applicant's part of DMF to the customers of API (drug products manufacturer) which may be filed by customer with the regulatory agency.

6. Preparing and submitting the LoA (letter of access/letter of authorization) to the API customers and regulatory agencies. LoA is the letter which authorizes the regulatory agency to review the DMF/ASMF of the API manufacturer against the NDA/ANDA/MAA of the API customers (formulators).

7. Preparing technical packages for existing/prospective customer for initial assessment of the API.

8. Filing annual/biannual/quinquennial reports (which contain list of changes to the DMF/ASMF/dossier) with the regulatory agencies.

9. Maintenance of the complete history of each API (filing history with agencies/customers, amendments, annual reports).

10. Taking part in the drugs development process by advising the R&D scientists regarding various guidelines, laws and regulations.

   Note: Apart from the above work profile there may be other responsibilities for regulatory affairs professionals too.

Job of a regulatory affairs professional in a finished product/formulation manufacturing company:

1. Filing a NDA/ANDA/MAA of drug products with regulatory agencies for getting marketing approval.

2. Assessing and filing supplements/amendments/variations to the information (which may be related to manufacture, control, stability studies, etc.) in NDA/ANDA/MAA with the regulatory agencies for prior approval or after their implementation. Major supplements/amendments are to be reported prior to their implementation while minor supplements/amendments may be reported annually. The classification of amendments will be dealt in the later posts.

3. Filing annual/biannual reports (which contain list of changes to the NDA/ANDA/MAA) with the regulatory agencies.

4. Reporting any adverse effects which have occurred/may occur due to the use drug products.

5. Maintenance of the complete history of each drug products (filing history with agencies/customers, amendments, annual reports).

6. Taking part in design and revision of drug product labels, packing leaflets.

7. Taking part in the formulation of development process by advising the R&D scientists regarding various guidelines, laws and regulations.

   Note: Apart from the above work profile there may be other responsibilities for regulatory affairs professionals too.

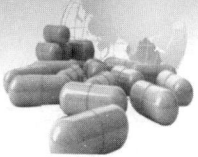

List of some common abbreviation and their full forms

S.No	Abbreviation	Full form
1.	NDA	New drug application
2.	ANDA	Abbreviated new drug application
3.	INDA	Investigational new drug application
4.	MAA	Marketing authorization application
5.	DMF	Drug master file
6.	ASMF	Active substance master file
7.	CEP	Certificate of suitability to the monograph of European Pharmacopoeia
8.	CGMP	Current good manufacturing practice
9.	ICH	The international conference on harmonization of technical requirements for registration of pharmaceuticals for human use
10.	GCP	Good clinical practice
11.	GLP	Good laboratory practice

Major Regulatory Authorities Worldwide

Some important drug regulatory authorities (across the world) are given below. Each and every country has its own regulatory authority. Some important authorities are mentioned in Table 1.1 along with their country name.

S.No	Country	Regulatory authority
		Table 1.1: List of regulatory authorities and country
1.	India	Central Drugs Standard Control Organization (CDSCO) Drugs Controller General of India (DCGI)
2.	US	Food and Drug Administration (US FDA)
3.	UK	Medicines and Health Care Products Regulatory Agency (MHRA)
4.	Australia	Therapeutic Goods Administration (TGA)
5.	Japan	Japanese Ministry of Health, Labor and Welfare (MHLW)
6.	Canada	Health Canada
7.	Brazil	Agency Nacional Degradation Vigilancia Sanitaria (ANVISA)
8.	South Africa	Medicines Contol Council (MCC)
9.	Europe	European Directorate for Quality of Medicines (EDQM), European Medicines Evaluation Agencies (EMEA)
10.	New Zealand	Medsafe—Medicines and Medical Devices Safety Authority

Contd.

	Table 1.2: List of regulatory authorities and country	*Contd.*
S.No	**Country**	**Regulatory authority**
11.	Singapore	Health and Science Authority (HSA)
12.	Malaysia	Drug Control Authority, National Pharmaceutical Control Bureau, Ministry of Health Malaysia, Biro Pengawalan Farmaseutikal Kebangsaan (BPFK)
13.	Philippines	Food and Drug Administration (FDA), Philippines
14.	China	CFDA→ China Food and Drug Administration.
15.	Nigeria	NAFDAC→ National Agency for Food and Drug Administration and Control
16.	Korea	KFDA→ Korea Food and Drug Administration
17.	Zimbabwe	MCAZ→ Medicine Control Authority of Zimbabwe
18.	Denmark	Denish Medical Agency
19.	Ireland	Irish Medical Agency
20.	Germany	Federal Institute for Drugs and Medical Devices
21.	Ukraine	Ministry of Health
22.	Uganda	Uganda National Council for Science and Technology (UNCST)
23.	Hong Kong	Department of Health: Pharmaceutical Services
24.	Paraguay	Ministry of Health

The drug regulatory affairs department plays an important role in the entire drug developments process. The drug development process is further explained in the following chapter. Right from the conceptualization till the launch of the product, the regulatory affairs department is involved. Even after approval, the regulatory affairs department plays an important role throughout the life cycle of the product by submission of annual reports, renewals, variations, PSURs, etc. So, the time by which the product is in market the regulatory affairs department has a role.

Looking into the current scenario, the role of RA department becomes more important. Day-by-day more regulations are coming up and regulatory approval process is becoming more and more stringent, hence need for the regulatory affairs professional is increasing.

ORGANIZATION AND FUNCTIONS OF KEY REGULATORY AGENCIES

US FDA

The Food and Drug Administration of the US has the responsibility for regulation of drugs and biological products which are manufactured and/or sold in the United States. The FDA is part of the Health and Human Service Department of the US Government. The organizational structure of the US FDA is mentioned in Fig. 1.3.

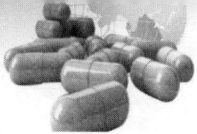
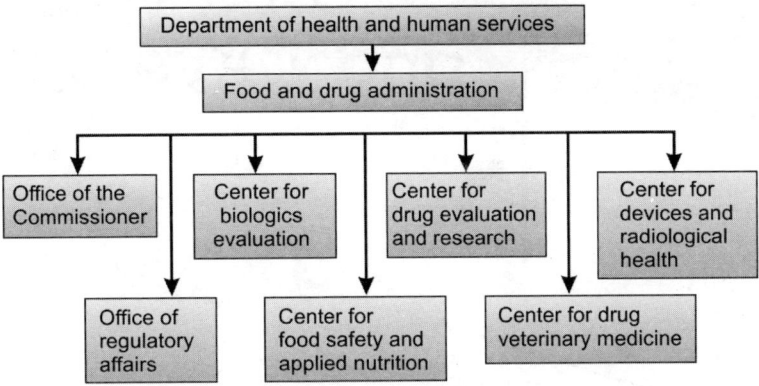

Fig. 1.3: The organizational structure of the US FDA

THE FEDERAL FOOD, DRUG AND COSMETIC (FDC) ACT OF 1938

Congress passed The Federal Food, Drug, and Cosmetic (FDC) Act of 1938, which requires that new drugs show safety before selling. This starts a new system of drug regulation and Act requires that safe limits be set for unavoidable poisonous matter and allows for factory inspections.

The Federal Trade Commission is given power to oversee advertising for all FDA-regulated products except prescription drugs.

FDA states that sulfanilamide and other dangerous drugs must be given under the direction of a medical expert. This begins the requirement for prescription only (non-narcotic) drugs. The Federal Food, Drug and Cosmetic Act is divided in to the below mentioned chapters (Table 1.2):

Table 1.2: Division of the Federal Food, Drug and Cosmetic Act	
Chapter One	Short title
Chapter Two	Definitions and terms
Chapter Three	Prohibited Acts and penalties, adulteration and misbranding, injunctive relief, strict liability standard (intent), due process, enforcement through justice department
Chapter Four	Authorizes the regulation of foods, standards of identity emergency permit controls
Chapter Five	Drugs and devices
Chapter Six	Cosmetics
Chapter Seven	Administrative provisions and tools, rule making, regulation promulgation, inspections
Chapter Eight	Imports and exports
Chapter Nine	Repeal of 1906 Act, exemptions (meats, biologics, etc.)

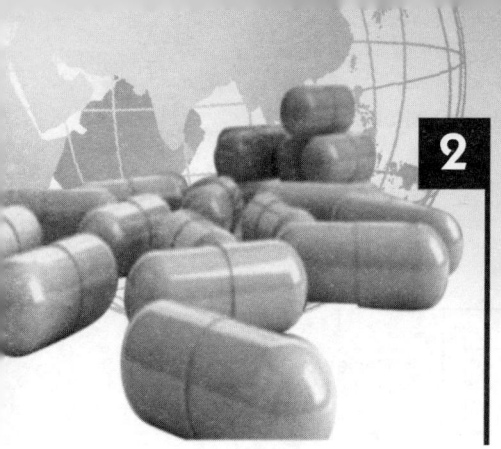

2

Drug Discovery and Development Process

The Drug Regulatory Authorities are responsible for assuring that foods and cosmetics are safe and that medicines and medical devices are both safe and effective. Balancing the efficacy and safety of these products is the core public health protection duty of the drug regulatory agencies. This goal requires examining efficacy as determined from well-controlled trials, effectiveness as determined from actual use in uncontrolled settings, and safety for both prescription and over-the-counter pharmaceuticals before approving a medication for market.

The purpose of this lesson is to present a concise overview of the drug approval process. It will briefly review the journey of a new product from early development until approval by the FDA for prescription use.

DRUG DISCOVERY AND DRUG DEVELOPMENT PROCESS

Drug discovery and drug development process of the US is generally divided into phases. The first is the preclinical phase, which usually takes 3 to 4 years to complete. If successful, this phase is followed by an application to the FDA as an investigational new drug (IND). After an IND is approved, the next steps are clinical phases 1, 2, and 3, which require approximately 1, 2, and 3 years, respectively, for completion. Importantly, throughout this process the FDA and investigators leading the trials communicate with each other so that issues such as safety are monitored. The manufacturer then files a new drug application (NDA) with the FDA for approval. This application can either be approved or rejected, or the FDA might request further study before making a decision. Overall, this entire process, on average, takes between 8 and 12 years (Fig. 2.1).

Birth of a Drug

The first step in the drug development process is the discovery of a new molecular entity (NME) to treat a targeted disease. The drug discovery process requires a significant amount of time and financial investment.

Preclinical: The first step, a preclinical phase, is to find a promising agent, which involves taking advantage of the advances made in understanding a disease, pharmacology, computer science, and chemistry. Breaking down a disease process

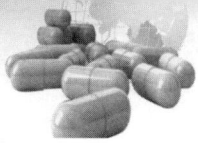

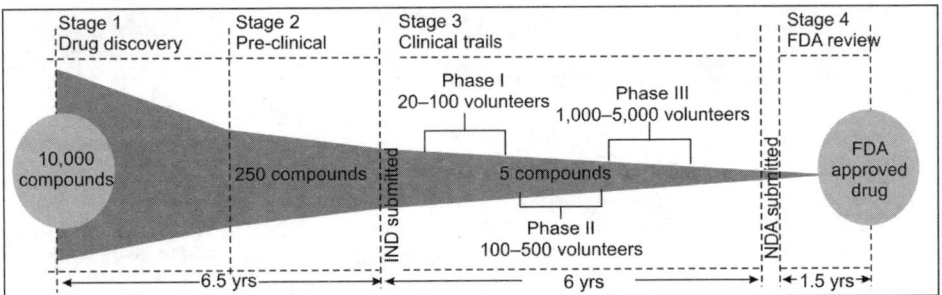

Fig. 2.1: Stage of drug discovery and drug development process of the US

into its components can provide clues for targeting drug development. For example, if an enzyme is determined to be a key component of a disease process, a researcher might seek ways to inhibit this enzyme. Advances in basic science might help by ascertaining the active enzyme site. Numerous compounds might be synthesized and tested before a promising agent emerges. Computer modeling often helps in selecting (or in selection of) what compounds might be the most promising.

Investigational New Drug (IND) Application (Preclinical Approval Process)

This application is submitted to the FDA after completion of preclinical studies. The IND contains the results of preclinical studies and describes how a drug will be evaluated in human subjects. The IND must be approved before human clinical trials can be conducted. The IND application includes chemical and manufacturing data, animal test results, including pharmacology and safety data, the rationale for testing a new compound in humans, strategies for protection of human volunteers, and a plan for clinical testing. If the FDA is satisfied with the documentation, the stage is set for phase 1 clinical trial (Fig. 2.2).

Clinical: The next step before attempting a clinical trial in humans is to test the drug in living animals, usually rodents. The FDA requires that certain animal tests should be conducted before humans are exposed to a new molecular entity. The objectives of early *in vivo* testing are to demonstrate the safety of the proposed medication. For example, tests should prove that the compound does not cause chromosomal damage and is not toxic at the doses that would most likely be effective. The results of these tests are used to support the IND application that is filed with the FDA. The IND application includes chemical and manufacturing data, animal test results, including pharmacology and safety data, the rationale for testing a new compound in humans, strategies for protection of human volunteers, and a plan for clinical testing. If the FDA is satisfied with the documentation, the stage is set for phase 1 clinical trials.

Phase 1 studies focus on the safety and pharmacology of a compound. During this stage, low doses of a compound are administered to a small group of healthy volunteers who are closely supervised. In cases of severe or life-threatening illnesses, volunteers with the disease may be used. Generally, 20 to 100 volunteers are enrolled in a phase 1 trial. These studies usually start with very low doses, which are

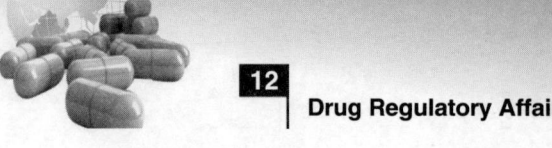

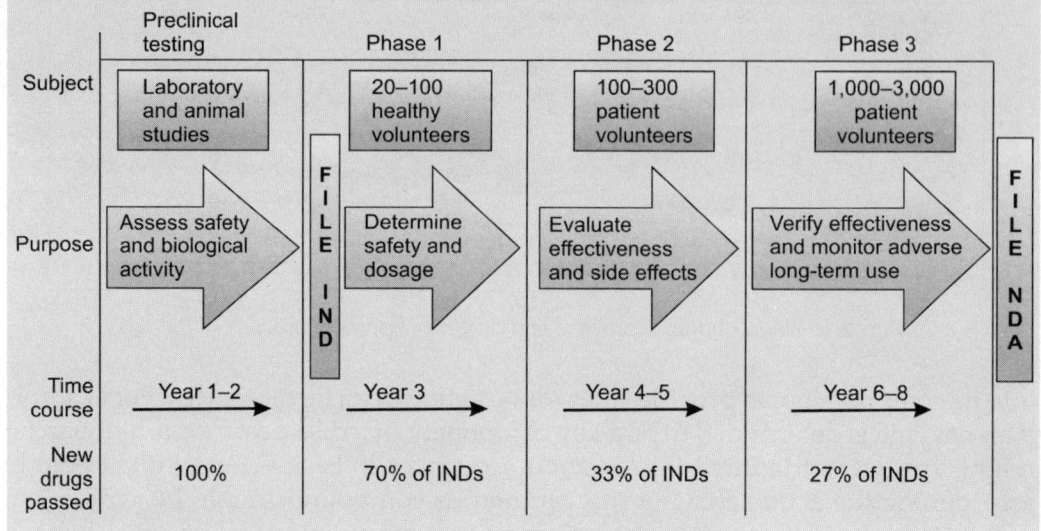

Fig. 2.2: Phases in drug discovery and drug development process of the US

gradually increased. On average, about two-thirds of phase 1 compounds are found safe enough to progress to phase 2.

Phase 2 studies examine the effectiveness of a compound. To avoid unnecessarily exposure of a human volunteer to a potentially harmful substance, studies are based on an analysis of the fewest volunteers needed to provide sufficient statistical power to determine efficacy. Typically, phase 2 studies involve 100 to 300 patients who suffer from the condition for which the new drug is intended to treat. During phase 2 studies, researchers seek to determine the effective dose, the method of delivery (e.g. oral or intravenous), and the dosing interval, as well as to reconfirm product safety. Patients in this stage are monitored carefully and assessed continuously. A substantial number of these drug trials are discontinued during phase 2 studies. Some drugs turn out to be ineffective, while others have safety problems or intolerable side effects.

Phase 3 trials are the final step before seeking FDA approval. During phase 3, researchers try to confirm previous findings in a larger population. These studies usually last from 2 to 10 years and involve thousands of patients across multiple sites. These studies are used to demonstrate further safety and effectiveness and to determine the best dosage. Despite the intense scrutiny, a product receives before undergoing expensive and extensive phase 3 testing, approximately 10% of medications fail in phase 3 trials.

NEW DRUG APPLICATION

If a drug survives the clinical trials, new drug application (NDA) is submitted to the FDA. An NDA contains all the preclinical and clinical information obtained during the testing phase. The application contains information on the chemical make-up and manufacturing process, pharmacology and toxicity of the compound,

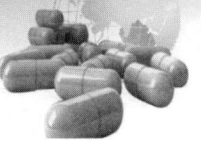

human pharmacokinetics, results of the clinical trials, and proposed labeling. An NDA can include experience with the medication from outside the United States as well as external studies related to the drug. An essential part of this process is the development of an appropriate dosage form (for example, tablets, capsules or injectables). The development of a dosage form moves in tandem with the clinical evaluation of the drug. Early formulations are used to establish therapeutic safety and efficacy. Commercial dosage formulations are developed as the NME enters phase II clinical trials. Scale-up to commercial manufacturing batch, sizes culminates in the manufacture of registration and validation batches to support regulatory filings and the launch of the commercial product.

Developing an appropriate dosage form, preparing necessary clinical trial materials and scaling-up the dosage form, manufacturing to commercial scale are all part of the development process. Through these activities, it must be demonstrated that the drug can be consistently manufactured at commercial batch sizes in accordance with applicable regulatory requirements. The data recorded during development activities are included in the chemistry, manufacturing and controls section of the required new drug application (NDA) for the FDA. A drug must meet regulatory requirements at all phases of the clinical trial and drug development processes or it will not be approved for human use. Figure 2.3 shows the phases of pharmaceutical development as they are related to the clinical trial approval process.

Pre-approval Inspection

Following the completion of the clinical trials, an NDA is submitted to the FDA for marketing approval. During the review process, a pre-approval inspection (PAI) is conducted on the manufacturing facility listed in the NDA for the commercial

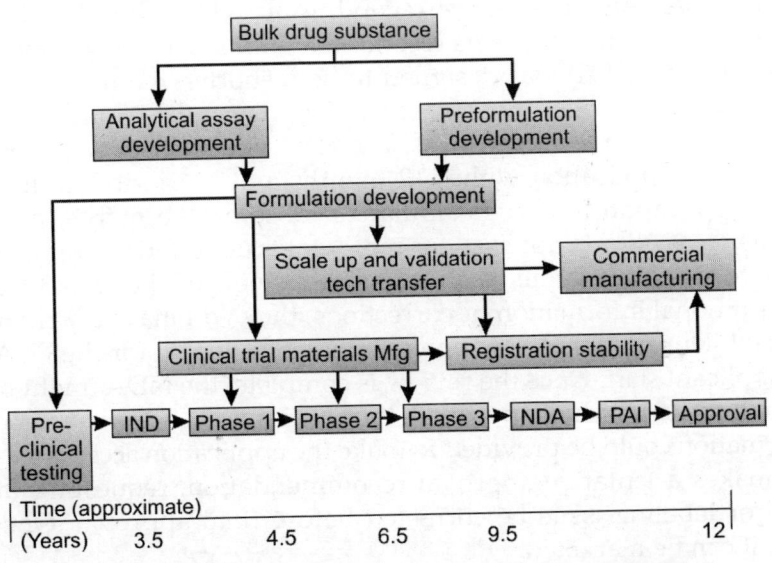

Fig. 2.3: Phases in pharmaceutical product development

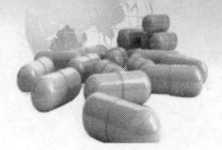

manufacturing of the new drug. Those portions of the facility involved in the manufacture of the new drug must be inspected for compliance with cGMP and approved before the new drug can be marketed. Upon approval, the new drug is available for physicians to prescribe.

Post-marketing Approval (Phase IV)

Some approvals contain conditions that must be met after initial marketing, such as conducting additional clinical studies. For example, the FDA might request a post-marketing, or phase 4, study to examine the risks and benefits of the new drug in a different population or to conduct special monitoring in a high-risk population. Alternatively, a phase 4 study might be initiated by the sponsor to assess such issues as the longer term effects of drug exposure, to optimize the dose for marketing, to evaluate the effects in pediatric patients, or to examine the effectiveness of the drug for additional indications. Post-marketing surveillance is important, because even the most well-designed phase 3 studies might not uncover every problem that could become apparent once a product is widely used. Furthermore, the new product might be more widely used by groups that might not have been well studied in the clinical trials, such as elderly patients. A crucial element in this process is that physicians report any untowards complications. The FDA has setup a medical reporting program called Med watch to track serious adverse events. The manufacturer must report adverse drug reactions at quarterly intervals for the first-3 years after approval, including a special report for any serious and unexpected adverse reactions.

COMMERCIAL MANUFACTURING

Commercial manufacturing in the pharmaceutical industry relates to the manufacturing and packaging of finished dosage forms of approved drug products destined for consumer use. After receiving an NDA, the FDA completes an independent review and makes its recommendations. The Prescription Drug User Fee Act of 1992 (PDUFA) was designed to help shorten the review time. This act allowed the agency to collect user fees from pharmaceutical companies as financial support to enhance the review process. The 1992 act specifies that the FDA reviews a standard drug application within 12 months and a priority application within 6 months. Application for drugs similar to those on the market are considered standard, whereas priority applications represent drugs offering important advances in addition to existing treatments. If during the review the FDA staff feels there is a need for additional information or corrections, they will make a written request to the applicant. During the review process it is not unusual for the FDA to interact with the applicant staff. Once the review is complete, the NDA might be approved or rejected. If the drug is not approved, the applicant is given the reasons why and what information could be provided to make the application acceptable. Sometimes the FDA makes a tentative approval recommendation, requesting that a minor deficiency or labeling issue be corrected before final approval. Once a drug is approved, it can be marketed.

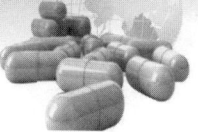

GENERIC DRUG DEVELOPMENT APPROVAL PROCESS

A generic drug product is one that is comparable to an innovator drug product in dosage form, strength, route of administration, quality, performance characteristics and intended use. All approved products, both innovator and generic, are listed in FDA's Approved Drug Products with Therapeutic Equivalence Evaluation (Orange Book). A generic drug is simply a copy of innovator/brand name drug and is bioequivalent to a brand name drug with respect to pharmacokinetic and pharmacodynamic properties. Generic medicines must contain the same active ingredient at the same strength as the innovator drug product and are required to meet the same pharmacopoeial standards. Therefore, generics are assumed identical in dose, strengh, route of administration, safety, efficacy and intended use.

An Abbreviated New Drug Application (ANDA) contains data which when submitted to FDA's Center for Drug Evaluation and Research, Office of Generic Drugs, provides for the review and ultimate approval of a generic drug product. Once approved, an applicant may manufacture and market the generic drug product to provide a safe, effective, low cost alternative to the public.

Generic drug applications are termed "abbreviated" because they are generally not required to include preclinical (animal) and clinical (human) data to establish safety and effectiveness. Instead, generic applicants must scientifically demonstrate that their product is bioequivalent (i.e. performs in the same manner as the innovator drug). One way scientists demonstrate bioequivalence is to measure the time it takes the generic drug to reach the bloodstream in 24 to 36 healthy, volunteers. This gives them the rate of absorption, or bioavailability, of the generic drug, which they can then compare to that of the innovator drug. The generic version must deliver the same amount of active ingredients into a patient's bloodstream in the same amount of time as the innovator drug.

Generic drugs are safe and effective alternatives to brand name drugs reduce the cost of prescription drugs for both consumers and the government, represent 70% of the total prescriptions dispensed in the US. In order to receive FDA approval, generic drugs must:

1. Contain the same active ingredient
2. Be the same strength
3. Be the same dosage form (tablet, capsule, etc.), and
4. Have the same route of administration (oral, topical, injectable, etc.) as the brand name drug.
5. In addition to being pharmaceutically equivalent, generic drugs must also be "bioequivalent" to the brand name drug. That means the generic drugs will work in the body in the same way (same amount goes into the body within the same time frame) and be as safe and effective as the brand name drug.

BRANDED VS GENERIC PRODUCT DEVELOPMENT

As stated earlier, that generic drug approval process does not require the generic drug manufacturer to repeat costly animal and clinical research on ingredients or

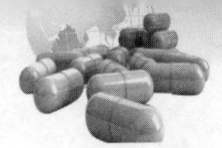

S. No.	NDA	ANDA
	NDA	*ANDA*
1.	Chemistry	Chemistry
2.	Manufacturing	Manufacturing
3.	Testing	Testing
4.	Labeling	Labeling
5.	Inspection	Inspection
6.	Animal studies Clinical studies Bioavailability	Bioequivalence studies

Table 2.1: NDA vs ANDA requirements: Regulatory data differences

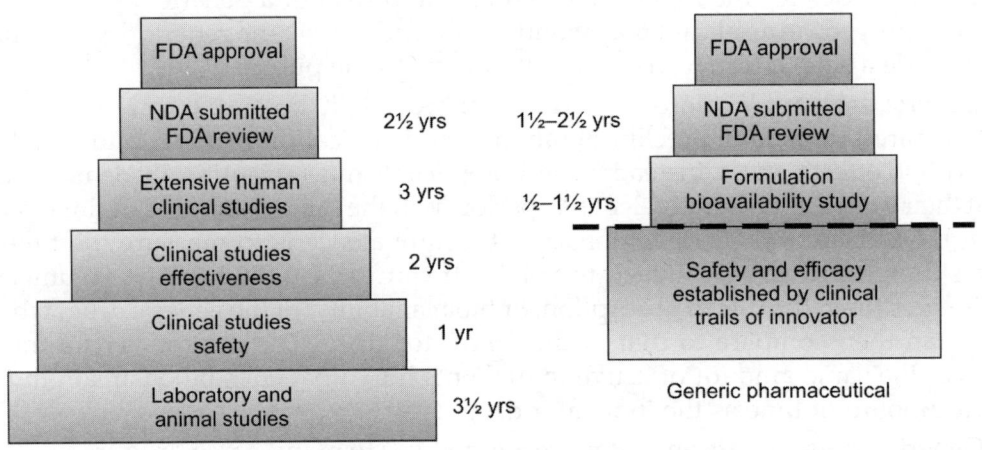

Fig. 2.4: Developmental stages in branded vs generic product development

dosage forms already approved for safety and effectiveness, manufacturer have to show only bioequivalence data (Table 2.1). Hence, generic drug development requires far less time (~ 3 years) in comparison to brand product development (~12 years), as depicted in Fig. 2.4.

The major differences are with respect to the:
1. Development of the active ingredient
2. Preclinical animal studies for safety and efficacy
3. Human clinical trials to prove the efficacy and safety of the active ingredient

COMPARISON OF INNOVATOR AND GENERIC DRUGS

Differences between generic and brand name drugs

A brand name drug is supplied by one company and sold under a trademarked name, e.g. Prilosec (Table 2.2). Generic drugs may be supplied by more than one

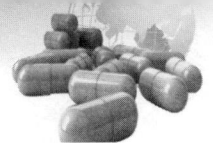

S. No.	Parameters	Innovator drug	Generic drug
	Table 2.2: Comparison of innovator and generic drugs		
1.	Active ingredients	Same	Same
2.	Safety and efficacy	Same	Same
3.	Quality and strength	Same	Same
4.	Performance and standards	Same	Same
5.	Costs/prescription	Highly expensive	Less expensive
6.	FDA inspection of manufacturing facilities	Yes	Yes
7.	FDA reviews reports of adverse reactions	Yes	Yes
8.	FDA reviews drug labeling	Yes	No
9.	Extensive research and development investments	Yes	No
10.	Expensive marketing and advertising	Yes	No
11.	Patent protection	Yes	No
12.	FDA review to show active ingredient is equivalent to original	—	Yes
13.	Product development time	~ 12 yrs	2– 4 yrs

company and sold under the name(s) of the active ingredient(s), e.g. omeprazole. Generic drugs are less expensive because it is not necessary to repeat:

I. Discovery

II. Preclinical studies

III. Clinical studies (repeating would be unethical)

The major components of an ANDA review include bioequivalence evaluation, chemistry/microbiologic evaluation, inspection of the manufacturing facility, and review of the proposed label.

BIOAVAILABILITY AND BIOEQUIVALENCE REQUIREMENTS FOR GENERIC DRUGS

With the passage of the 1984 Drug Price Competition and Patent Term Restoration Amendments to Food, Drug and Cosmetic Act, bioequivalence took on added importance for generic drugs. As defined in implementing regulations, an applicant submitting an Abbreviated New Drug Application under section 505(j) of the Act (except Suitability Petitions submitted under 505(j)(2)(c) of the Act) must demonstrate both pharmaceutical equivalence (PE) and bioequivalence (BE) between generic product and listed innovator reference drug product. With acceptance of this documentation by FDA, along with other information, the generic product is deemed bioequivalent, therapeutically equivalent and interchangeable with the listed reference drug product.

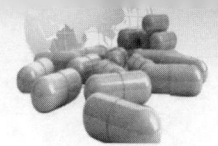

The term bioavailability is most commonly applied to oral dosage forms and refers to the rate and the extent to which the drug is absorbed from the GIT into the systemic circulation. Other routes of administration designed to deliver the drug to the blood such as the transdermal, rectal, buccal routes and inhalation can also be subject to the bioequivalence studies. The purpose of bioequivalence study is to compare the bioavailabilities of the generic (test) and brand (reference) product.

Each subject's drug or metabolite concentration-time profile is examined to determine the maximum concentration (C_{max}), the time at the C_{max} is observed (T_{max}), and the area under the concentration-time curve (AUC) the last measurable concentration. In addition, the AUC to infinity (AUC infinity) is computed from the last measurable concentration and the calculated elimination rate-constant.

ORANGE BOOK

The publication, *Approved Drug Products with Therapeutic Equivalence Evaluations* (the list, commonly known as the Orange Book), identify drug products approved on the basis of safety and effectiveness by the food and drug administration (FDA) under the Federal Food, Drug, and Cosmetic Act (the Act).

Drugs on the market approved only on the basis of safety (covered by the ongoing drug efficacy study implementation [DESI] review). The main criterion for the inclusion of any product is that the product is the subject of an application with an effective approval that has not been withdrawn for safety or efficacy reasons. Inclusion of products on the list is independent of any current regulatory action through administrative or judicial means against a drug product. In addition, the list contains therapeutic equivalence evaluations for approved multisource prescription drug products.

The list was distributed as a proposal in January 1979. It included only currently marketed prescription drug products approved by FDA through new drug applications (NDAs) and abbreviated new drug applications (ANDAs) under the provisions of Section 505 of the Act.

The list is composed of four parts:

1. Approved prescription drug products with therapeutic equivalence evaluations;
2. Approved over-the-counter (OTC) drug products for those drugs that may not be marketed without NDAs or ANDAs because they are not covered under existing OTC monographs;
3. Drug products with approval under Section 505 of the Act administered by the Center for Biologics Evaluation and Research; and
4. A cumulative list of approved products that have never been marketed, are for exportation, are for military use, have been discontinued from marketing, or have had their approvals withdrawn for other than safety or efficacy reasons subsequent to being discontinued from marketing. [**Note:** Newly approved products are added to parts 1, 2, or 3 of the list, depending on the dispensing requirements (prescription or OTC) or approval authority, unless the Orange Book staff is otherwise notified before publication.]

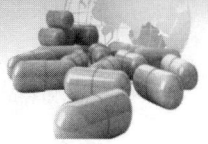
Under the 1984 Amendments, some drug products are given tentative approvals. The agency will not include drug products with tentative approval in the list; however, they are available at ANDA approvals. When the tentative approval becomes a full approval through a subsequent action letter to the application holder, the agency will list the drug product and the final approval date in the appropriate approved drug product list.

Therapeutic Equivalence-related Terms

Pharmaceutical equivalents. Drug products are considered pharmaceutical equivalents, if they contain the same active ingredient(s), are of the same dosage form, route of administration and are identical in strength or concentration (e.g. chlordiazepoxide hydrochloride, 5 mg capsules). Pharmaceutically equivalent drug products are formulated to contain the same amount of active ingredient in the same dosage form and to meet the same or compendial or other applicable standards (i.e. strength, quality, purity, and identity), but they may differ in characteristics such as shape, scoring configuration, release mechanisms, packaging, excipients (including colors, flavors, preservatives), expiration time, and, within certain limits, labeling.

Pharmaceutical alternatives. Drug products are considered pharmaceutical alternatives if they contain the same therapeutic moiety, but are different salts, esters, or complexes of that moiety, or are different dosage forms or strengths (e.g. tetracycline hydrochloride, 250 mg capsules vs. tetracycline phosphate complex, 250 mg capsules; quinidine sulfate, 200 mg tablets vs. quinidine sulfate, 200 mg capsules). Data are generally not available for FDA to make the determination of tablet to capsule bioequivalence. Different dosage forms and strengths within a product line by a single manufacturer are thus pharmaceutical alternatives, as are extended-release products when compared with immediate-release or standard-release formulations of the same active ingredient.

Therapeutic equivalents. Drug products are considered to be therapeutic equivalents only if they are pharmaceutical equivalents and if they can be expected to have the same clinical effect and safety profile when administered to patients under the conditions specified in the labeling.

FDA classifies as therapeutically equivalent those products that meet the following general criteria: (1) they are approved as safe and effective; (2) they are pharmaceutical equivalents in that they (a) contain identical amounts of the same active drug ingredient in the same dosage form and route of administration, and (b) meet compendial or other applicable standards of strength, quality, purity, and identity; (3) they are bioequivalent in that (a) they do not present a known or potential bioequivalence problem, and they meet an acceptable *in vitro* standard, or (b) if they do present such a known or potential problem, they are shown to meet an appropriate bioequivalence standard; (4) they are adequately labeled; (5) they are manufactured in compliance with current good manufacturing practice regulations. The concept of therapeutic equivalence, as used to develop the list, applies only to drug products containing the same active ingredient(s) and does not encompass a comparison of different therapeutic agents used for the same condition (e.g. ibuprofen vs naproxen

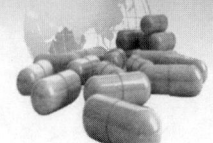

for the treatment of pain). Any drug product in the list repackaged and/or distributed by other than the application holder is considered to be therapeutically equivalent to the application holder's drug product even if the application holder's drug product is single source or coded as non-equivalent (e.g. BN). Also, distributors or repackagers of an application holder's drug product are considered to have the same code as the application holder. Therapeutic equivalence determinations are not made for unapproved, off-label indications.

FDA considers drug products to be therapeutically equivalent if they meet the criteria outlined above, even though they may differ in certain other characteristics such as shape, scoring configuration, release mechanisms, packaging, excipients (including colors, flavors, preservatives), expiration date/time and minor aspects of labeling (e.g. the presence of specific pharmacokinetic information) and storage conditions. When such differences are important in the care of a particular patient, it may be appropriate for the prescribing physician to require that a particular brand be dispensed as a medical necessity. With this limitation, however, FDA believes that products classified as therapeutically equivalent can be substituted with the full expectation that the substituted product will produce the same clinical effect and safety profile as the prescribed product.

Bioavailability. This term means the rate and extent to which the active ingredient or active moiety is absorbed from a drug product and becomes available at the site of action. For drug products that are not intended to be absorbed into the bloodstream, bioavailability may be assessed by measurements intended to reflect the rate and extent to which the active ingredient or active moiety becomes available at the site of action.

Bioequivalent drug products. This term describes pharmaceutical equivalent or alternative products that display comparable bioavailability when studied under similar experimental conditions. Section 505 (j)(8)(B) of the Act describes one set of conditions under which a test and reference listed drug shall be considered bioequivalent: the rate and extent of absorption of the test drug do not show a significant difference from the rate and extent of absorption of the reference drug when administered at the same molar dose of the therapeutic ingredient under similar experimental conditions in either a single dose or multiple doses; or the extent of absorption of the test drug does not show a significant difference from the extent of absorption of the reference drug when administered at the same molar dose of the therapeutic ingredient under similar experimental conditions in either a single dose or multiple doses and the difference from the reference drug in the rate of absorption of the drug is intentional, is reflected in its proposed labeling, is not essential to the attainment of effective body drugs concentrations on chronic use, and is considered medically insignificant for the drug.

Where these above methods are not applicable (e.g. for drug products that are not intended to be absorbed into the bloodstream), other *in vivo* or *in vitro* test methods to demonstrate bioequivalence may be appropriate.

Bioequivalence may sometimes be demonstrated using an *in vitro* bioequivalence standard, especially when such an *in vitro* test has been correlated with human *in*

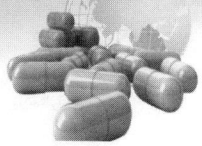

vivo bioavailability data. In other situations, bioequivalence may sometimes be demonstrated through comparative clinical trials or pharmacodynamic studies.

Reference Listed Drug

A reference listed drug (RLD) (21 CFR 314.94(a)(3)) means the listed drug identified by FDA as the drug product upon which an applicant relies in seeking approval of its ANDA.

FDA has identified in the prescription drug product and OTC drug product lists those reference listed drugs to which the *in vivo* bioequivalence (reference standard) and, in some instances, the *in vitro* bioequivalence of the applicant's product is compared. By designating a single reference listed drug as the standard to which all generic versions must be shown to be bioequivalent, FDA hopes to avoid possible significant variations among generic drugs and their brand name counterpart. Such variations could result if generic drugs were compared to different reference listed drugs. However, in some instances when listed drugs are approved for a single drug product, a product not designated as the reference listed drug and not shown to be bioequivalent to the reference listed drug may be shielded from generic competition. A firm wishing to market a generic version of a listed drug that is not designated as the reference listed drug may petition the Agency through the citizen petition procedure (see 21 CFR 10.25(a) and CFR 10.30). When the citizen petition is approved, the second listed drug will be designated as an additional reference listed drug and the petitioner may submit an abbreviated new drug application citing the designated reference listed drug.

Products meeting necessary bioequivalence requirements explain the *AB, AB1, AB2, AB3* coding system for multisource drug products listed under the same heading with two reference listed drugs.

In addition, there are two situations in which two listed drugs that have been shown to be bioequivalent to each other may both be designated as reference listed drugs. The first situation occurs when the *in vivo* determination of bioequivalence is self-evident and a waiver of the *in vitro* methodology. The reference listed drug is identified by the symbol "+" in the prescription and over-the-counter (OTC) drug product lists. These identified reference listed drugs represent the best judgment of the division of bioequivalence at this time. The prescription and OTC drug product lists identify reference drugs for oral dosage forms, injectables, ophthalmics, otics, and topical products. It is recommended that a firm planning to conduct an *in vivo* waiver of bioequivalence will be requested, contact the Division of bioequivalence, office of generic drugs, to confirm the appropriate reference listed drug.

Multisource and single-source drug products. FDA has evaluated for therapeutic equivalence only multisource prescription drug products approved under Section 505 of the Act, which in most instances means those pharmaceutical equivalents available from more than one manufacturer. For such products, a therapeutic equivalence code is included and, in addition, product information is highlighted

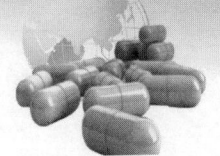

in bold face and underlined. Those products with approved applications that are single-source (i.e. there is only one approved product available for that active ingredient, dosage form, route of administration, and strength) are also included on the list, but no therapeutic equivalence code is included with such products. Any drug product in the list repackaged and/or distributed by other than the application holder is considered to be therapeutically equivalent to the application holder's drug product even if the application holder's drug product is single source or coded as non-equivalent (e.g. BN). Also, although not identified in the list, distributors or repackagers of an application holder's drug product are considered to have the same code as the application holder. The details of these codes and the policies underlying them are discussed in Therapeutic Equivalence Evaluations Codes.

Products on the list are identified by the names of the holders of approved applications (applicants) who may not necessarily be the manufacturer of the product. The applicant may have had its product manufactured by a contract manufacturer and may simply be distributing the product for which it has obtained approval. In most instances, however, the manufacturer of the product is also the applicant. The name of the manufacturer is permitted by regulation to appear on the label, even when the manufacturer is not the marketer.

Therapeutic Equivalence Evaluations Codes

The coding system for therapeutic equivalence evaluations is constructed to allow users to determine quickly whether the agency has evaluated a particular approved product as therapeutically equivalent to other pharmaceutically equivalent products (first letter) and to provide additional information on the basis of FDA's evaluations (second letter). With a few exceptions, the therapeutic equivalence evaluation date is the same as the approval date.

The two basic categories into which multisource drugs have been placed are indicated by the first letter as follows:

A Drug product that FDA consider to be therapeutically equivalent to other pharmaceutically equivalent products, i.e. drug products for which:

1. There are no known or suspected bioequivalence problems. These are designated AA, AN, AO, AP, or AT, depending on the dosage form; or

2. Actual or potential bioequivalence problems have been resolved with adequate *in vivo* and/or *in vitro* evidence supporting bioequivalence. These are designated AB.

B Drug product that FDA at this time, consider NOT to be therapeutically equivalent to other pharmaceutically equivalent products, i.e. drug products for which actual or potential bioequivalence problems have not been resolved by adequate evidence of bioequivalence. Often the problem is with specific dosage forms rather than with the active ingredients. These are designated BC, BD, BE, BN, BP, BR, BS, BT, BX, or B.

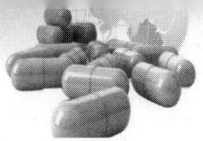

Individual drug products have been evaluated as therapeutically equivalent to the reference product in accordance with the definitions and policies outlined below:

"A" CODES

Drug products that are considered to be therapeutically equivalent to other pharmaceutically equivalent products.

"A" products are those for which actual or potential bioequivalence problems have been resolved with adequate *in vivo* and/or *in vitro* evidence supporting bioequivalence. Drug products designated with an "A" code fall under one of two main policies:

1. For those active ingredients or dosage forms for which no *in vivo* bioequivalence issue is known or suspected, the information necessary to show bioequivalence between pharmaceutically equivalent products is presumed and considered self-evident based on other data in the application for some dosage forms (e.g. solutions) or satisfied for solid oral dosage forms by a showing that an acceptable *in vitro* dissolution standard is met. A therapeutically equivalent rating is assigned such products so long as they are manufactured in accordance with current good manufacturing practice regulations and meet the other requirements of their approved applications (these are designated AA, AN, AO, AP, or AT, depending on the dosage form, as described below); or

2. For those DESI drug products containing active ingredients or dosage forms that have been identified by FDA as having actual or potential bioequivalence problems, and for post-1962 drug products in a dosage form presenting a potential bioequivalence problem, an evaluation of therapeutic equivalence is assigned to pharmaceutical equivalents only if the approved application contains adequate scientific evidence establishing through *in vivo* and/or *in vitro* studies the bioequivalence of the product to a selected reference product (these products are designated as AB).

There are some general principles that may affect the substitution of pharmaceutically equivalent products in specific cases. Prescribers and dispensers of drugs should be alert to these principles so as to deal appropriately with situations that require professional judgment and discretion.

There may be labeling differences among pharmaceutically equivalent products that require attention on the part of the health professional. For example, pharmaceutically equivalent powders to be reconstituted for administration as oral or injectable liquids may vary with respect to their expiration time or storage conditions after reconstitution. An FDA evaluation that such products are therapeutically equivalent is applicable only when each product is reconstituted, stored, and used under the conditions specified in the labeling of that product.

The specific sub-codes for those drugs evaluated as therapeutically equivalent and the policies underlying these sub-codes follow:

AA products in conventional dosage forms not presenting bioequivalence problems.

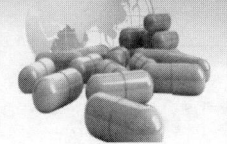

Products coded as **AA** contain active ingredients and dosage forms that are not regarded as presenting either actual or potential bioequivalence problems or drug quality or standards issues. However, all oral dosage forms must, nonetheless, meet an appropriate *in vitro* bioequivalence standard that is acceptable to the agency in order to be approved.

AB, AB1, AB2, AB3 ... products meeting necessary bioequivalence requirements

Multisource drug products listed under the same heading (i.e. identical active ingredients(s), dosage form, and route(s) of administration) and having the same strength (see **Therapeutic Equivalence-related Terms, Pharmaceutical Equivalents)** generally will be coded AB if a study is submitted demonstrating bioequivalence.

In certain instances, a number is added to the end of the AB code to make a three character code (i.e. AB1, AB2, AB3, etc.). Three-character codes are assigned only in situations when more than one reference listed drug of the same strength has been designated under the same heading. Two or more reference listed drugs are generally selected only when there are at least two potential reference drug products which are not bioequivalent to each other. If a study is submitted that demonstrates bioequivalence to a specific listed drug product, the generic product will be given the same three-character code as the reference listed drug it was compared against. For example, Adalat® CC (Miles) and Procardia XL® (Pfizer), extended-release tablets, are listed under the active ingredient nifedipine. These drug products, listed under the same heading, are not bioequivalent to each other. Generic drug products deemed by FDA to be bioequivalent to Adalat® CC and Procardia XL® have been approved, Adalat® CC and Procardia XL® have been assigned ratings of AB1 and AB2, respectively. The generic drug products bioequivalent to Adalat® CC would be assigned a rating of AB1 and those bioequivalent to Procardia XL® would be assigned a rating of AB2. (The assignment of an AB1 or AB2 rating to a specific product does not imply product preference.) Even though drug products of distributors and/or repackagers are not included in the list, they are considered therapeutically equivalent to the application holder's drug product if the application holder's drug product is rated either with an AB or three-character code or is single source in the list. Drugs coded as AB under a heading are considered therapeutically equivalent only to other drugs coded as AB under that heading. Drugs coded with a three-character code under a heading are considered therapeutically equivalent only to other drugs coded with the same three-character code under that heading.

AN Solutions and Powders for Aerosolization

Uncertainty regarding the therapeutic equivalence of aerosolized products arises primarily because of differences in the drug delivery system. Solutions and powders intended for aerosolization that are marketed for use in any of several delivery systems are considered to be pharmaceutically and therapeutically equivalent and are coded AN. Those products that are compatible only with a specific delivery system or those products that are packaged in and with a specific delivery system are coded BN, unless they have met an appropriate bioequivalence standard. Solutions or

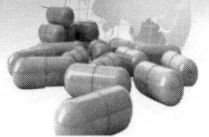

suspensions in a specific delivery system will be coded AN if the bioequivalence standard is based upon *in vitro* methodology, if bioequivalence needs to be demonstrated by *in vivo* methodology then the drug products will be coded AB.

AO Injectable Oil Solutions

The absorption of drugs in injectable (parenteral) oil solutions may vary substantially with the type of oil employed as a vehicle and the concentration of the active ingredient. Injectable oil solutions are therefore considered to be pharmaceutically and therapeutically equivalent only when the active ingredient, its concentration, and the type of oil used as a vehicle are all identical.

AP injectable aqueous solutions, and in certain instances, intravenous non-aqueous solutions

It should be noted that even though injectable (parenteral) products under a specific listing may be evaluated as therapeutically equivalent, there may be important differences among the products in the general category, **Injectable; Injection**. For example, some injectable products that are rated therapeutically equivalent are labeled for different routes of administration. In addition, some products evaluated as therapeutically equivalent may have different preservatives or no preservatives at all. Injectable products available as dry powders for reconstitution, concentrated sterile solutions for dilution, or sterile solutions ready for injection are pharmaceutical alternative drug products. They are not rated as therapeutically equivalent (AP) to each other even if these pharmaceutical alternative drug products are designed to produce the same concentration prior to injection and are similarly labeled. Consistent with accepted professional practice, it is the responsibility of the prescriber, dispenser, or individual administering the product to be familiar with a product's labeling to assure that it is given only by the route(s) of administration stated in the labeling.

Certain commonly used large volume intravenous products in glass containers are not included on the list (e.g. dextrose injection 5%, dextrose injection 10%, sodium chloride injection 0.9%) since these products are on the market without FDA approval and the FDA has not published conditions for marketing such parenteral products under approved NDAs. When packaged in plastic containers, however, FDA regulations require approved applications prior to marketing. Approval then depends on, among other things, the extent of the available safety data involving the specific plastic component of the product. All large volume parenteral products are manufactured under similar standards, regardless of whether they are packaged in glass or plastic. Thus, FDA has no reason to believe that the packaging container of large volume parenteral drug products that are pharmaceutically equivalent would have any effect on their therapeutic equivalence.

The strength of parenteral drugs products is defined as the total drug content of the container. Until recently the strength of liquid parenteral drug products in the Orange Book have not been displayed. The concentration of the liquid parenteral drug product in the Orange Book has been shown as xmg/ml. The amount of dry

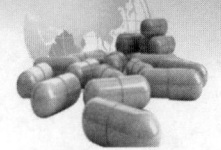

powder or freeze dried powder in a container has always been identified as the strength.

With the finalization of the Waxman-Hatch amendments that characterized each strength of a drug product as a listed drug it became evident that the format of the Orange Book should be changed to reflect each strength of a parenteral solution. To this end the OGD has started to display the strength of all new approvals of parenteral solutions. Previously we would have displayed only the concentration of an approved parenteral solution, e.g. 50 mg/ml. If this drug product had a 20 ml and 60 ml container approved the two products would be shown as 1 gm/20 ml (50 mg/ml) and 3 gm/ 60 ml (50 mg/ml).

AT Topical Products

There are a variety of topical dosage forms available for dermatologic, ophthalmic, otic, rectal, and vaginal administration, including creams, gels, lotions, oils, ointments, pastes, solutions, sprays and suppositories. Even though different topical dosage forms may contain the same active ingredient and potency, these dosage forms are not considered pharmaceutically equivalent. Therefore, they are not considered therapeutically equivalent. All solutions and DESI drug products containing the same active ingredient in the same topical dosage form for which a waiver of *in vivo* bioequivalence has been granted and for which chemistry and manufacturing processes are adequate to demonstrate bioequivalence, are considered therapeutically equivalent and coded AT. Pharmaceutically equivalent topical products that raise questions of bioequivalence, including all post-1962 non-solution topical drug products, are coded AB when supported by adequate bioequivalence data, and BT in the absence of such data.

"B" CODES

Drug products that FDA, at this time, considers not to be therapeutically equivalent to other pharmaceutically equivalent products.

"B" products, for which actual or potential bioequivalence problems have not been resolved by adequate evidence of bioequivalence, often have a problem with specific dosage forms rather than with the active ingredients. Drug products designated with a "B" code fall under one of three main policies:

1. The drug products are contain active ingredients or manufactured in dosage forms that have been identified by the agency as having documented bioequivalence problems or a significant potential for such problems and for which no adequate studies demonstrating bioequivalence have been submitted to FDA; or
2. The quality standards are inadequate or FDA has an insufficient basis to determine therapeutic equivalence; or
3. The drug products are under regulatory review.

The specific coding definitions and policies for the "B" sub-codes are as follows:

B Drug products requiring further FDA investigation and review to determine therapeutic equivalence.

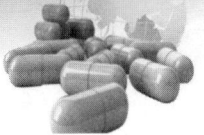

The code B is assigned to products previously assigned an A or B code when FDA receives new information that raises a significant question regarding therapeutic equivalence that can be resolved only through further agency investigation and/or review of data and information submitted by the applicant. The B code signifies that the agency will take no position regarding the therapeutic equivalence of the product until the agency completes its investigation and review.

BC extended-release dosage forms (capsules, injectables and tablets)

Extended-release tablets are formulated in such a manner as to make the contained medicament available over an extended period of time after ingestion.

Although bioavailability studies have been conducted on these dosage forms, they may be subject to bioavailability differences, primarily because firms developing extended-release products for the same active ingredient rarely employ the same formulation approach. FDA, therefore, does not consider different extended-release dosage forms containing the same active ingredient in equal strength to be therapeutically equivalent unless equivalence between individual products in both rate and extent has been specifically demonstrated through appropriate bioequivalence studies. Extended-release products for which such bioequivalence data have not been submitted are coded BC, while those for which such data are available have been coded AB.

BD active ingredients and dosage forms with documented bioequivalence problems

The BD code denotes products containing active ingredients with known bioequivalence problems and for which adequate studies have not been submitted to FDA demonstrating bioequivalence. Where studies showing bioequivalence have been submitted, the product has been coded AB.

BE delayed-release oral dosage forms

Where the drug may be destroyed or inactivated by the gastric juice or where it may irritate the gastric mucosa, the use of "enteric" coatings is indicated. Such coatings are intended to delay the release of the medication until the tablet has passed through the stomach. Drug products in delayed-release dosage forms containing the same active ingredients are subject to significant differences in absorption. Unless otherwise specifically noted, the agency considers different delayed-release products containing the same active ingredients as presenting a potential bioequivalence problem and codes these products BE in the absence of *in vivo* studies showing bioequivalence. If adequate *in vivo* studies have demonstrated the bioequivalence of specific delayed-release products, such products are coded AB.

BN products in aerosol-nebulizer drug delivery systems

This code applies to drug solutions or powders that are marketed only as a component of, or as compatible with, a specific drug delivery system. There may, for example, be significant differences in the dose of drug and particle size delivered by different products of this type. Therefore, the agency does not consider different

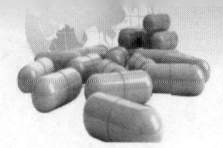

metered aerosol dosage forms containing the same active ingredient(s) in equal strengths to be therapeutically equivalent unless the drug products meet an appropriate bioequivalence standard, such products are coded AB.

BP active ingredients and dosage forms with potential bioequivalence problems

FDA's bioequivalence regulations (21 CFR 320.33) contain criteria and procedures for determining whether a specific active ingredient in a specific dosage form has a potential for causing a bioequivalence problem. It is FDA's policy to consider an ingredient meeting these criteria as having a potential bioequivalence problem even in the absence of positive data demonstrating inequivalence. Pharmaceutically equivalent products containing these ingredients in oral dosage forms are coded BP until adequate *in vivo* bioequivalence data are submitted, such products are coded AB. Injectable suspensions containing an active ingredient suspended in an aqueous or oleaginous vehicle have also been coded BP. Injectable suspensions are subject to bioequivalence problems because differences in particle size, polymorphic structure of the suspended active ingredient, or the suspension formulation can significantly affect the rate of release and absorption. FDA does not consider pharmaceutical equivalents of these products bioequivalent without adequate evidence of bioequivalence, such products would be coded AB.

BR suppositories or enemas that deliver drugs for systemic absorption

The absorption of active ingredients from suppositories or enemas that are intended to have a systemic effect (as distinct from suppositories administered for local effect) can vary significantly from product to product. Therefore, FDA considers pharmaceutically equivalent systemic suppositories or enemas bioequivalent only if *in vivo* evidence of bioequivalence is available. In those cases where *in vivo* evidence is available, the product is coded AB. If such evidence is not available, the products are coded BR.

BS products having drug standard deficiencies

If the drug standards for an active ingredient in a particular dosage form are found by FDA to be deficient so as to prevent an FDA evaluation of either pharmaceutical or therapeutic equivalence, all drug products containing that active ingredient in that dosage form are coded BS. For example, if the standards permit a wide variation in pharmacologically active components of the active ingredient such that pharmaceutical equivalence is in question, all products containing that active ingredient in that dosage form are coded BS.

BT topical products with bioequivalence issues

This code applies mainly to post-1962 dermatologic, ophthalmic, otic, rectal, and vaginal products for topical administration, including creams, ointments, gels, lotions, pastes, and sprays, as well as suppositories not intended for systemic drug absorption. Topical products evaluated as having acceptable clinical performance, but that are not bioequivalent to other pharmaceutically equivalent products or that lack sufficient evidence of bioequivalence, will be coded BT.

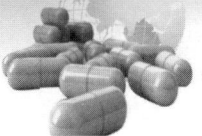

BX drug products for which the data are insufficient to determine therapeutic equivalence

The code BX is assigned to specific drug products for which the data that have been reviewed by the agency are insufficient to determine therapeutic equivalence under the policies stated in this document. In these situations, the drug products are presumed to be therapeutically in equivalent until the agency has determined that there is adequate information to make a full evaluation of therapeutic equivalence.

AUTHORIZED GENERICS (PSEUDO-GENERICS)

In accordance with the Drug Price Competition and Patent Term Restoration Act (Hatch-Waxman), generic pharmaceutical manufacturers who successfully challenge (via paragraph IV certification included in the ANDAs) patents covering branded pharmaceuticals before the brands' patents expire receive 180 days exclusivity in which they were free to market their generic product without competition from other generics approved after the first date of submission as ANDAs. During this time, generic manufacturer(s) could penetrate the market without the lower price that would be likely with more generic competitors. After the 180 days exclusivity period, more generic versions of the drug are typically launched. Revisions made in MMA of 2003 were designed in part to promote more competition among generics during the 180 days exclusivity period.

"An authorized generic is defined by the FDA as "*Any marketing by an NDA holder or authorized by an NDA holder, including through a third-party distributor, of the drug product approved under the NDA in a manner equivalent to the marketing practices of holders of an approved ANDA for that drug*".

The practice of authorizing generics allows the holder of the NDA to market a competing product, during the 180 days exclusivity period of the first-to-file Paragraph IV challenger(s). Authorized generic agreements predominantly come in one of 2 forms. The branded manufacturer with the NDA can either license its product to a generic pharmaceutical company (licensees have included a range of generic companies, including generic industry leaders such as Barr, Andrx, Mylan and Teva); or the brand manufacturer can market the product through an in-house generic subsidiary.

The introduction of a pseudo-generic into the market before any independent generic enters, while costly to the brand manufacturer, is correlated with higher prices of the branded product than if the brand manufacturer delayed entry of the pseudo-generic by several months. One argument in favor of pseudo-generics is that when they enter early, they may lead to cost savings for buyers—consumers, insurers, and governments.

DRUG PRICE COMPETITION AND PATENT TERM RESTORATION ACT OF 1984

Introduction

Drug Price Competition and Patent Term Restoration Act of 1984 is commonly called as Hatch-Waxman Act. "The Hatch-Waxman Act is an act dealing with the

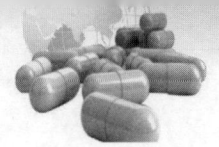

approval of generic drugs and associated conditions for getting their approval from FDA, market exclusivity, rights of exclusivity, patent term extension and Orange Book listing".

The act was necessitated by the following observations:

Absence of generic drug manufacturing: Sometime in the year 1962 it was observed in the USA that out of the 150 off patent drugs in the market, there were no generic drugs. Owing to cumbersome procedures involved, manufacturers were simply not interested to take up manufacture of these, even though these were cheaper.

Cumbersome regulatory procedures: Many companies did not go in for manufacture of generic drugs because of the impractical and nonscientific manner in which the regulatory authorities viewed the approval process and insisted upon proving the obvious.

Patients were denied the option of cheaper drugs: Owing to the cumbersome procedures involved, drug companies did not want to waste time and money on clinical trials of generic drugs, insisted upon by regulatory authorities.

"The Hatch-Waxman Act is an act dealing with the approval of generic drugs and associated conditions for getting their approval from the Food and Drug Administration (FDA), market exclusivity, rights of exclusivity, patent term extension and Orange Book Listing" .

The dual purposes of the Hatch-Waxman Act were to encourage the development of new innovator drugs by extending patent rights and to establish procedures facilitating the approval of low-cost generic drugs. These amendments to the Food, Drug and Cosmetics Act codified in statute an abbreviated process (ANDA) for post-1962 drugs whereby a generic company could gain approval of its version of a drug without repeating the expensive and lengthy clinical trials used to establish safety and efficacy of the innovator drug. Under certain circumstances relating to patent challenges, the first generic version of a brand-name innovator medication receives a 180 days period of market exclusivity.

General Provisions of the Act

Maintaining list of patents which would be infringed: Each holder of an approved new drug application (NDA) must list pertinent patents it believes would be infringed if a generic drug were marketed before expiration of these patents. The FDA maintains a list of such patents in its publication, Approved Drug Products with Therapeutic Equivalence Evaluations (commonly known as Orange Book).

Only bioavailability studies and not clinical trials needed for approval: FDA can only ask for bioavailability studies in respect of an ANDA and not for clinical trials, etc. (For bioavailability FDA uses the + 20% test, i.e. the amount of active ingredient in the blood serum over a period of time has to come within + 20% of that which is observed with the patented drug.)

Patent certification scheme (Para I, II, III and IV certifications): While filing an ANDA, a generic firm must certify any one of the following:

i. Patent information on the drug has not been filed (in the Orange Book).

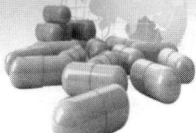

ii. Patent has already expired.

iii. Date on which patent will expire, and that the generic drug will not go to the market until that date passes.

iv. Patent is invalid and will not be infringed by the manufacture, use or sale of the generic drug. This last certification is known as a paragraph IV certification. The applicant filing through para IV certification gets 180 days market exclusivity as reward for challenging innovator company i.e. patent litigation.

The above certifications are also called paragraph I, II, III and IV certifications. In case of certification I and II, approval for manufacture can be granted immediately. In case of III, approval for ANDA can be made effective from the date of patent expiration. In case of IV, it is mandatory for the manufacturer to notify the original patent holder, who can take up to 45 days to bring an infringement suit against the manufacturer; if he feels his intellectual property rights (IPRs) are being violated. However, if no such action is taken within the stipulated period, certification of the ANDA applicant will be accepted by the FDA.

If an infringement action is brought in time, FDA must suspend approval of the ANDA until the date of court's decision. If the court decision goes in favor of the patent owner, FDA will suspend the approval till expiry of the patent. FDA does not wait indefinitely—the maximum time available for coming to a decision is 30 months (2.5 years) after the expiry of 45 days.

The first generic applicant to file paragraph IV certification is awarded a 180 days (6 months) market exclusivity period by the FDA. The six month exclusivity period will start at the earliest of the two dates-the date of commencement of commercial marketing of the generics or the day a court decides that the patent which is the subject matter of Para IV certification, is invalid or not infringed.

The 180 days exclusivity period granted to the first generic applicant would become available to the next-filed applicant if the first applicant reached a financial settlement with the brand name to stay out of the market until the patents have expired; fails to go to market within 90 days once their application is effective; does not get FDA approval within 30 months; fails to challenge a new patent within 60 days; withdraws their application; or is determined by the Health and Human Services Secretary to have engaged in anti-competitive activities.

Data exclusivity period for NMEs: New molecular entities approved by the FDA will enjoy data exclusivity for a period of 5 years from the date of approval of the NME by the FDA. A generic version cannot be approved during these five years.

Data exclusivity period for supplements: Supplements requiring clinical trials will enjoy 3 years data exclusivity period.

Extension of the original patent term: Original patent term can be extended by a maximum of five years, if undue delays take place during the regulatory process (FDA approval).

The "Bolar" Provision

America's Hatch-Waxman legislation included a section, now known as the "Bolar provision", that allowed the importation of the small amount of raw material

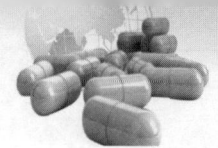

required to prepare the compound and test a product before a patent expired. This permitted a generic company to complete its FDA application prior to patent expiration so that the generic version would be available for marketing immediately a patent expired. This provision was a *sine qua non* for generic negotiators of the legislation, since 99% of the raw materials for generic production in the United States are imported.

Changes to the Hatch-Waxman Act

Under the Medicare Prescription Drug and Modernization Act of 2003, some changes have been made in the existing Hatch-Waxman Act. These are as follows:

Non-extension of the 30 months period

As per modified rules, only one 30 months stay will be permitted in case of those patents listed in the Orange Book, when an ANDA is filed under paragraph IV certification. Modifications to the 30 months stay are allowed based on district court judgments. Patent holders included new patents in the Orange Book after receiving notification regarding Para IV certification and thus extended the 30 months period.

Time limit for informing patent owner

The company filing ANDA under Para IV must submit full and complete information over and above what is necessary under current law and must notify the patent owner within 20 days.

Provision for allowing declaratory judgment

If patent owner does not file infringement proceeding within 45 days of notification issued by ANDA applicant, the applicant may request for a declaratory judgment and thus avoid being sued. If sued, applicant may file a counter claim requiring patent owner to make changes in the orange book listings. This favors the patent holder, because he does not have to pay any damages for not modifying the Orange Book listing in time and there is apparently no time limit for making such modifications.

Benefit of exclusivity for several ANDAs filed on same day allowed

It is now possible for many generic companies to qualify for the 180 days market exclusivity if several ANDAs are filed on the same day.

The Consequences of the Hatch-Waxman Act

The positive effects

The Act seems to have achieved its purpose in many respects. Generic drug availability is on the rise. There has been an increase in the percentage of branded drugs that have a generic competitor on the market—nearly 100% of the top-selling drugs with expired patents have generic versions, compared to only 36% in 1983, and generic share of prescription drug volume has increased by almost 150% since 1984.

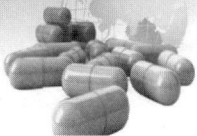

The negative effects

However, many pharmaceutical companies have used the incentives for challenging invalid patents through the 180 days exclusivity period, and compensate innovator drug companies wishing to defend their intellectual property patents by the grant of the 30 months stay of ANDA approvals during patent litigation; some would call them loopholes to actually extend exclusivity periods and block competition from entering the market.

The most common means of twisting Hatch-Waxman into a vehicle for Big Pharma to extend exclusivity is through patent litigation. Recall that if the patent holder sues a paragraph IV ANDA filer within 45 days of being notified of the certification, the FDA will not even consider any application related to the drug in question for thirty months, essentially granting the patent holder an additional two and a half years of marketing exclusivity. This encourages a present NDA holder to file suit every time any generic files a paragraph IV certification, even if the suit would be frivolous, since regardless of the merits of the suit the FDA must automatically grant the stay, blocking all generic competition.

A closely related potential for abuse is the 6 months of exclusivity granted to the first paragraph IV ANDA filer. The exclusivity for a generic version only begins when either the patent infringement litigation is finally adjudicated, or upon the commencement of marketing by the generic. Therefore, if litigants settle the suit out of court, the only mechanism to trigger starting the clock on the 180-day exclusivity is the marketing of the generic product. This situation has led to cases where brand name companies (the patent holder) pay the generic company (the alleged infringer) to defer or abandon marketing generics pursuant to the settlement agreement. Therefore, this exclusivity grant under the Hatch-Waxman Act meant as an incentive to the generic, can actually be a backdoor method of restraining competition by keeping generic products out of the marketplace indefinitely.

The Prescription Drug User Fee Act

The Prescription Drug User Fee Act (PDUFA), enacted in 1992 and renewed in 1997 (PDUFA II) and 2002 (PDUFA III) authorizes FDA to collect fees from companies that produce certain human drug and biological products. PDUFA established three types of user fees—application fees, establishment fees, and product fees. Since the passage of PDUFA, user fees have played an important role in expediting the drug approval process.

Generic Drug User Fee Amendments of 2012

The US Food and Drug Administration (FDA) published its guidance for industry on the Generic Drug User Fee Amendments (GDUFA) of 2012 in a question-and-answer format. This guidance provides answers to anticipated questions regarding GDUFA, specifically on the topics of fees, self-identification of facilities, sites and organizations, review of generic drug submissions, and inspections and compliance, a summary of which is found in the guidance document. A failure to pay a required fee may result in a refusal to receive an Abbreviated New Drug Application (ANDA) or any supplement to an ANDA, or in a drug being deemed misbranded.

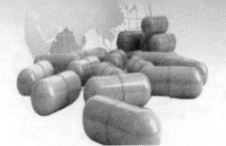

Backlog fee: Each person who owns an original ANDA pending on October 1, 2012 that has not been withdrawn, tentatively approved, or approved by September 28, 2012 will be required to pay a backlog fee. The FDA will determine the backlog fee by dividing $50 million by the number of original ANDAs pending on October 1, 2012. The backlog fee is a one-time fee for each pending original ANDA. To avoid this backlog fee, written notification of a withdrawal of an original ANDA must be received by September 28, 2012. Failure to pay the backlog fee will place the person on a "publicly available arrears list, and FDA will not receive a new ANDA or supplement submitted by that person, or any affiliate . . . of that person".

Drug master file (DMF) fee: Only DMFs for a Type II API will incur the one-time DMF fee. The fee is incurred on the date the first generic drug submission references the DMF by initial letter of authorization (if that DMF has not previously been relied upon) on or after October 1, 2012, except for Fiscal Year 2013 when the fee will be due not "earlier than 30 days after publication of the final DMF fee in the **Federal Register** or 30 days after enactment of an appropriations Act that provides for the collection and obligation of generic drug user fees, whichever is later". The fee is required regardless of whether the DMF has been reviewed prior to GDUFA implementation. The FDA estimates that the DMF fee will be about $43,000. DMF holders, however, may pay the fee prior to any request for a letter of authorization. An ANDA applicant may also pay this fee. A DMF will be "deemed not available for reference" for failure to pay the DMF fee. If such fee is not received within 20 calendar days of notification of failure to pay, any "ANDA referencing the DMF will not be received".

ANDA and prior approval supplement (PAS) fees: The FDA estimates that the ANDA fee will be about $53,000 and the PAS fee will be about $27,000. These fees are incurred at the time of submission, except for Fiscal Year 2013 when "fees will not be due earlier than 30 days after publication of the ANDA and PAS fees in the **Federal Register** or 30 days after enactment of an appropriations Act that provides for the collection and obligation of generic drug user fees, whichever is later". If an application is refused for reasons other than failure to pay fees, a partial refund of 75 percent of the fee will be accorded to the applicant. The FDA will not receive any ANDA or PAS if the fee is not paid within 20 calendar days of the due date. Additionally, any active pharmaceutical ingredient (API) manufactured by the applicant will require the payment of a one-time API-related fee for each API. The API-related fee "is a function of the number of APIs referenced in the application and the number of facilities in which those APIs are manufactured. If the ANDA references more than one facility as manufacturing each API, the applicant must pay the API-related fee for each such facility".

Facility fees: Finished dosage form (FDF) and API facilities fees will be "determined after the self-identification process." Self-identification is required for (1) facilities that manufacture, or intend to manufacture, human generic drug APIs and/or FDFs; (2) sites that package the FDF; (3) sites that are identified in a generic drug submission that subdivide the contents of the primary container/closure system; (4) bioequivalence/bioavailability sites that conduct clinical testing, bioanalytical testing, and/or *in vitro* testing; and (5) sites that perform testing of one or more attributes/

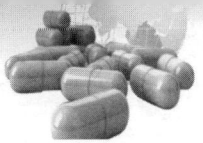

characteristics of the FDF or API. However, only facilities that manufacture, or intend to manufacture, generic drug APIs or FDFs, or both, are required to pay facility fees". If a company manufactures such products in different geographic locations, in facilities under the control of multiple management entities, or in separate buildings that are not "within close proximity ... and are capable of being inspected by the FDA during a single inspection" each facility must be separately identified. Any FDFs or APIs manufactured in a facility that is not self-identified will be deemed misbranded and will violate federal law if shipped in interstate commerce or imported into the US. The fees for each identified FDF or API facility will be determined after completion of the self-identification process and, for Fiscal Year 2013, "will be due within 45 days after publication of the final facility fee amounts in the **Federal Register**, or 30 days after the enactment of an appropriations Act providing for the collection and obligation of generic drug user fees, whichever is later". Thereafter, the annual fee "will be due on the first business day on or after October 1 of each fiscal year, or the first business day after the enactment of an appropriations Act that provides for the collection and obligation of fees". For foreign facilities, the fee "shall not be less than $15,000 and not more than $30,000 higher than the amount of the fee for a domestic facility" and "will be set on the basis of the FDA's estimate of the average direct cost differential between foreign inspections and domestic inspections". If the facility fee is not paid, "no new generic drug submission referencing the facility will be received", "the facility will be placed on a publicly available arrears list if the fee is not fully paid within 20 days of the due date", and "all FDFs or APIs manufactured in the non-paying facility and all FDFs containing APIs manufactured in such a facility will be deemed misbranded".

Supplemental New Drug Approval Process (SNDA)

Manufacturer of new drug applications (NDAs) and abbreviated new drug applications (ANDAs) who intend to make postapproval changes can do so in accordance with section 506A of the Federal Food, Drug, and Cosmetic Act (the Act) and § 314.70 (21 CFR 314.70). Post-approval changes can be categorized and applied in below mentioned categories:

1. Components and composition,
2. Manufacturing sites,
3. Manufacturing process,
4. Specifications,
5. Container closure system, and
6. Labeling, as well as
7. Miscellaneous changes, and
8. Multiple related changes.

Section 506A of the Act and § 314.70 provide for four reporting categories as mentioned below:

A *major change* is a change that has a substantial potential to have an adverse effect on the identity, strength, quality, purity, or potency of a drug product as

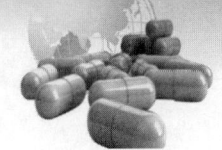

these factors may relate to the safety or effectiveness of the drug product. A major change requires the submission of a supplement and approval by FDA prior to distribution of the drug product made using the change. This type of supplement is called, and should be clearly labeled, a *prior approval supplement* (§ 314.70(b)). An applicant may ask FDA to expedite its review of a prior approval supplement for public health reasons (e.g. drug shortage) or if a delay in making the change of described in it would impose an extraordinary hardship on the applicant. This type of supplement is called, and should be clearly labeled, a *prior approval supplement-expedited review requested* (§ 314.70(b)(4)).FDA is most likely to grant requests for expedited review based on extraordinary hardship for manufacturing changes made necessary by catastrophic events (e.g. fire) or by events that could not be reasonably foreseen and for which the applicant could not plan.

A *moderate change* is a change that has a moderate potential to have an adverse effect on the identity, strength, quality, purity, or potency of the drug product as these factors may relate to the safety or effectiveness of the drug product. There are two types of moderate change. One type of moderate change requires the submission of a supplement to FDA at least 30 days before the distribution of the drug product made using the change. This type of supplement is called, and should be clearly labeled, a *supplement-changes being effected in 30 days* (§ 314.70(c)(3)). The drug product made using a moderate change cannot be distributed if FDA informs the applicant within 30 days of receipt of the supplement that a prior approval supplement is required (§ 314.70(c)(5)(i)). For each change, the supplement must contain information determined by FDA to be appropriate and must include the information developed by the applicant in assessing the effects of the change (§ 314.70(a)(2) and (c)(4)). If FDA informs the applicant within 30 days of receipt of the supplement that information is missing, distribution must be delayed until the supplement has been amended to provide the missing information (§ 314.70(c) (5)(ii)).

FDA may identify certain moderate changes for which distribution can occur when FDA receives the supplement (§ 314.70(c)(6)). This type of supplement is called, and should be clearly labeled, a *supplement changes-being-effected*. If, after review, FDA disapproves a changes-being-effected in 30 days supplement or changes-being-effected supplement, FDA may order the manufacturer to cease distribution of the drug products made using the disapproved change (§ 314.70(c)(7)).

A *minor change* is a change that has minimal potential to have an adverse effect on the identity, strength, quality, purity, or potency of the drug product as these factors may relate to the safety or effectiveness of the drug product. The applicant must describe minor changes in its next *Annual Report* (§ 314.70(d)).

The FDA has issued guidance document on scale-up post-approval changes (SUPAC). SUPAC is most significant guidance issued by US FDA and help this guidance is greatly welcomed by the industry because gives a very clear and straight idea for handling the post approval changes and greatly reduces the approval timeline.

Dosage forms covered under the SUPAC guidelines are mentioned below:

1. Immediate release (IR) solid oral dosage form

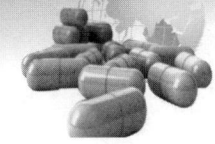

2. Modified release (MR) solid oral dosage forms, i.e. extended release, delayed release
3. Non-sterile semi-solid (SS) dosage forms, i.e. creams, ointments, suspensions, emulsions, gels and lotions.

Levels of change defined under SUPAC

1. **Level 1:** Unlikely to have impact on the product. Filed as an annual report update, normal testing as filed in NDA.
2. **Level 2:** Moderate changes such as technical grade of inert, filed as CBE or PA, accelerated stability and dissolution profile testing in addition to filed NDA.
3. **Level 3:** Likely to have impact, filed PA, stability and testing as above in addition a biostudy or *in vivo* correlation.

The SUPAC guidance mainly provides the guidance (though not the complete list, but some important aspects) on below mentioned changes:

a. Manufacturing site change
b. Batch size change
c. Manufacturing process change
d. Manufacturing equipment change
e. Analytical testing site change
f. Packaging site change
g. Component and composition—non-release controlling excipient
h. Component and composition—release controlling excipient

DRUG MASTER FILES

Introduction

A drug master file (DMF) is a voluntary submission to the Food and Drug Administration (FDA) that may be used to provide confidential detailed information about facilities, processes, or articles used in the manufacturing, processing, packaging, and storing of one or more human drugs. DMFs usually cover the chemistry, manufacturing and controls (CMC) of a component of a drug product e.g. drug substance, excipient, packaging material. Drug product information or non-CMC information may be filed in DMF.

The submission of a DMF is not required by law or FDA regulation. A DMF is submitted solely at the discretion of the holder. The information contained in the DMF may be used to support an investigational new drug application (IND), a new drug application (NDA), an abbreviated new drug application (ANDA), another DMF, an export application, or amendments and supplements to any of these.

A DMF is NOT a substitute for an IND, NDA, ANDA, or export application. It is not approved or disapproved. Technical contents of a DMF are reviewed only in connection with the review of an IND, NDA, ANDA, or an export application.

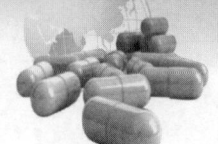

Drug master files (DMFs) are generally created to allow a party other than the holder of the DMF to reference material without disclosing to that party the contents of the file. When an applicant references its own material, the applicant should reference the information contained in its own IND, NDA, or ANDA directly rather than establishing a new DMF.

Types of Drug Master Files (DMFs)

There are five types of DMFs:

Type I—manufacturing site, facilities, operating procedures, and personnel

Type II—drug substance, drug substance intermediate, and material used in their preparation, or drug product

Type III—packaging material

Type IV—excipient, colorant, flavor, essence, or material used in their preparation

Type V—FDA accepted reference information

Type I: *Manufacturing site, facilities, operating procedures, and personnel*

A Type I DMF is recommended for a person outside of the United States to assist FDA in conducting on site inspections of their manufacturing facilities. The DMF should describe the manufacturing site, equipment capabilities, and operational layout.

A Type I DMF is normally not needed to describe domestic facilities, except in special cases, such as when a person is not registered and not routinely inspected.

The description of the site should include acreage, actual site address, and a map showing its location with respect to the nearest city. An aerial photograph and a diagram of the site may be helpful.

A diagram of major production and processing areas is helpful for understanding the operational layout. Major equipment should be described in terms of capabilities, application, and location. Make and model would not normally be needed unless the equipment is new or unique.

A diagram of major corporate organizational elements, with key manufacturing, quality control, and quality assurance positions highlighted, at both the manufacturing site and corporate headquarters, is also helpful.

Type II: *Drug substance, drug substance intermediate, and material used in their preparation, or drug product*

A Type II DMF should, in general, be limited to a single drug intermediate, drug substance, drug product, or type of material used in their preparation.

Drug substance intermediates, drug substances, and material used in their preparation

Summarize all significant steps in the manufacturing and controls of the drug intermediate or substance. Detailed guidance on what should be included in a

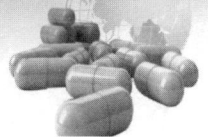

Type II DMF for drug substances and intermediates may be found in the following guidelines:

Drug Product

Manufacturing procedures and controls for finished dosage forms should ordinarily be submitted in an IND, NDA, ANDA, or export application. If this information cannot be submitted in an IND, NDA, ANDA, or export application, it should be submitted in a DMF. When a Type II DMF is submitted for a drug product, the applicant/sponsor should follow the guidance provided in the following guidelines:

Type III: *Packaging material*

Each packaging material should be identified by the intended use, components, composition, and controls for its release. The names of the suppliers or fabricators of the components used in preparing the packaging material and the acceptance specifications should also be given. Data supporting the acceptability of the packaging material for its intended use should also be submitted as outlined in the **"Guideline for submitting documentation for packaging for human drugs and biologics"**.

Toxicological data on these materials would be included under this type of DMF, if not otherwise available by cross reference to another document.

Type IV: *Excipient, colorant, flavor, essence, or material used in their preparation*

Each additive should be identified and characterized by its method of manufacture, release specifications, and testing methods.

Toxicological data on these materials would be included under this type of DMF, if not otherwise available by cross reference to another document.

Usually, the official compendia and FDA regulations for color additives (21 CFR Parts 70 through 82), direct food additives (21 CFR Parts 170 through 173), indirect food additives (21 CFR Parts 174 through 178), and food substances (21 CFR Parts 181 through 186) may be used as sources for release tests, specifications, and safety. Guidelines suggested for a Type II DMF may be helpful for preparing a Type IV DMF. The DMF should include any other supporting information and data that are not available by cross reference to another document.

Type V: *FDA accepted reference information*

FDA discourages the use of Type V DMFs for miscellaneous information, duplicate information, or information that should be included in one of the other types of DMFs. If any holder wishes to submit information and supporting data in a DMF that is not covered by Types I through IV, a holder must first submit a letter of intent to the Drug Master File Staff (for address, see D.5.a. of this Section). FDA will then contact the holder to discuss the proposed submission. Each DMF should contain only one type of information and all supporting data.

SUBMISSIONS TO DRUG MASTER FILES

Each DMF submission should contain a transmittal letter, administrative information about the submission, and the specific information to be included in the DMF as described in this section.

Original submissions of DMF includes:

a. Identification of submission: Original, the type of DMF as mentioned above and it's subject etc.
b. Identification of the applications, if known, that the DMF is intended to support, including the name and address of each sponsor, applicant, or holder, and all relevant document numbers.
c. Signature of the holder or the authorized representative.
d. Typewritten name and title of the signer.

Amendment submissions of DMF include:

a. Identification of submission: Amendment, the DMF number, type of DMF, and the subject of the amendment.
b. A description of the purpose of submission, e.g. update, revised formula, or revised process.
c. Signature of the holder or the authorized representative.
d. Typewritten name and title of the signer.

Administrative information

Administrative information should include the following:

Original submissions

a. Names and addresses of the following:
    1. DMF holder
    2. Corporate headquarters
    3. Manufacturing/processing facility
    4. Contact for FDA correspondence
    5. Agent(s), if any
b. The specific responsibilities of each person listed in any of the categories in Section a.
c. Statement of commitment.

   A signed statement by the holder certifying that the DMF is current and that the DMF holder will comply with the statements made in it.

Amendments

a. Name of DMF holder
b. DMF number
c. Name and address for correspondence
d. Affected section and/or page numbers of the DMF

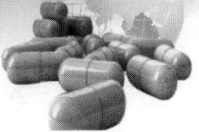

e. The name and address of each person whose IND, NDA, ANDA, DMF, or export application relies on the subject of the amendment for support.

f. The number of each IND, NDA, ANDA, DMF, and export application that relies on the subject of the amendment for support, if known.

g. Particular items within the IND, NDA, ANDA, DMF, and export application that are affected, if known.

Environmental assessment

Type II, Type III, and Type IV DMFs should contain a commitment by the firm that its facilities will be operated in compliance with applicable environmental laws. If a completed environmental assessment is needed, see 21 CFR Part 25.

Stability

Stability study design, data, interpretation, and other information should be submitted, when applicable.

Common Technical Document (CTD)

Module 1 administrative information that applies to DMFs

There are no forms for DMFs.

Section 1.2: Cover letter and statement of commitment

Section 1.3: Administrative information

1.3.1 Contact/sponsor/applicant information

1.3.1.1 Change of address or corporate name: Can be used to supply addresses of DMF holder and manufacturing and testing facilities

1.3.1.2 Change in contact/agent: Can be used to supply the name and address of contact persons and/or agents, including agent appointment letter.

1.4.1 Letter of authorization: Submission by the owner of information, giving authorization for the information to be used by another.

1.4.2 Statement of right of reference: Submission by recipient of a letter of authorization with a copy of the LOA and statement of right of reference (submitted in application or DMF that references a DMF).

1.4.3 List of authorized persons to incorporate by reference: Submitted in DMF annual reports.

Section 1.12.14 Environmental analysis

Module 2 Quality overall summary (QOS) expected to be submitted.

• 3.2.S Body of data for drug substance

• 3.2.R Regional information:executed batch records: At least one sample batch record (in English) is expected for drug substances and drug products.

Method validation package: Not usually submitted for DMFs. Complete methods validation information should be included in 3.2.S.4.3

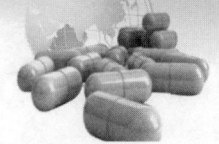

Letter of Authorization

The DMF will be reviewed only when it is referenced in an application or other DMF.

An letter of authorization (LOA) does two things:

1. Grants FDA authorization to review the DMF
2. Grants the authorized party the right to incorporate the information in the DMF by reference.

Mechanism to trigger the review of DMF:

The holder must submit an LOA (2 copies) to the DMF, then send a copy to the applicant. Applicant submits copy of LOA in their application. This is the mechanism to trigger review of the DMF.

Review of the DMF

DMFs are neither approved nor disapproved. A DMF is reviewed to determine whether it is adequate to support the particular application that references it. The DMF is reviewed using same regulatory and scientific criteria as review of application.

a. If more information is needed to complete the review a list of the information needed is communicated to the holder. The applicant is notified that information has been requested for the DMF. The letter to the applicant is either an information request (IR) or a complete response (CR) letter. The nature of the information requested is not communicated to the applicant.
b. If no information needed for DMF then no letter to DMF holder.

IR and CR Letters to Applicant

a. Not strictly a DMF issue but this affects how responses are dealt with the applicant.
b. IR letter to applicant: Review clock for NDA is not stopped. Responses may be reviewed at reviewer's discretion depending on timing relative to the due date.
c. CR letter to applicant: Review clock is stopped. Application (and supporting DMFs) will be reviewed only when all issues in CR letter (including DMF deficiencies) have been addressed.

Bulk Activities Post-approval Changes

Bulk activities post-approval changes (BACPAC) is an another important document issued by the FDA to provide guidance an post-approval changes in bulk active substances. This guidance document provide recommendations to bulk drug manufacturers who intend, during the post-approval to change the

1. Site of manufacture
2. Scale of manufacture
3. Equipment

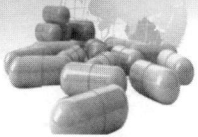

4. Specifications
5. Manufacturing process of intermediates

Post-marketing surveillance

Post-marketing drug surveillance refers to the monitoring of drugs once they reach the market after clinical trials. It evaluates drugs taken by individuals under a wide range of circumstances over an extended period of time. Such surveillance is much more likely to detect previously unrecognized positive or negative effects that may be associated with a drug. The majority of postmarketing surveillance concern adverse drug reactions (ADRs) monitoring and evaluation.

Benefits of post-marketing monitoring: Post-marketing studies has the ability to study the following:

1. Low frequency reactions (not identified in clinical trials)
2. High risk groups
3. Long-term effects
4. Drug/food interactions
5. Increased severity and/or reporting frequency of known reactions

Regulatory requirements for product approvals biological drug products: Biological drug products in US are regulated by the Center for Biologic Evaluation and Research (CBER). CBER is the center within FDA that regulates biological products for human use under applicable federal laws, including the Public Health Service Act and the Federal Food, Drug and Cosmetic Act. CBER protects and advances the public health by ensuring that biological products are safe and effective and available to those who need them. CBER also provides the public with information to promote the safe and appropriate use of biological products.

The Center for Biologics Evaluation and Research (CBER) regulates biological products under the authority of Section 351 of the Public Health Service Act. The task of CBER is to ensure the safety, effectiveness and timely delivery to patients of biological products through innovative regulations. CBER's review of new biological products, and for new indications for already approved products, requires evaluating scientific and clinical data submitted by manufacturers to determine whether the product meets CBER's standards for approval. After a thorough assessment of the data, CBER makes a decision based on the risk-benefit for the intended population and the product's intended use.

CBER regulates allergenics, blood and blood components, devices developed to prevent contamination of blood, blood components and cellular product, software used to collect blood and blood, gene therapy, human tissues, cellular products, vaccines, and xenotransplantation products (live animal organs, cells or tissues used to treat human diseases.

The CDER has responsibility for regulating monoclonal antibodies for use *in vivo*, proteins extracted from plants, animals or microorganisms, and other non-vaccine therapeutic immunotherapies. While it has some similarities to a New Drug Application (NDA), a BLA has its own unique set of requirements.

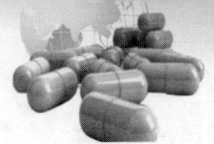

A biologics license application contains details on the chemistry, pharmacology, source materials, manufacturing processes, labeling and medical affects of the biologic product as well as data from clinical studies. If the information provided meets FDA requirements, the application is approved and a license is issued allowing the firm to market the product.

Biologic License Application Process

Biologic license application (BLA) is request for permission to introduce, or deliver for introduction, a biologic product into interstate commerce. (21 CFR 601.2) after the clinical trials are over.

In general terms the BLA consists of reports of all investigations sponsored by applicant and other information pertinent to an evaluation of the product's safety, effectiveness and purity.

Contents of BLA: A typical BLA contains following information:

1. Form FDA 356(h) (coversheet).
2. Applicant information.
3. Product/manufacturing information.
4. Preclinical studies.
5. Clinical studies.
6. Labeling information.

Form FDA 356(h)(coversheet):

Following information has to be submitted along with this form:

1. Applicant information: includes name, address of applicant and facilities and in case of foreign manufacturer then name and address of authorized agent.
2. Product/manufacturing information: includes information on raw material and its source; facility information and information about manufacturing process and formulation information.
3. Application information: as in whether the application is original (to be submitted by new applicant), amendment (to include information sought by FDA), resubmission (in response to a complete review letter), etc.

BLA safety, efficacy and use information—includes information on:

1. Preclinical studies.
2. Clinical studies:
    i. Phase 1 studies are safety and immunogenecity studies performed in a small number of closely monitored subjects.
    ii. Phase 2 studies are dose-ranging studies and may enroll hundreds of subjects.
    iii. Phase 3 studies typically enroll thousands of individuals and provide critical documentation of effectiveness and important additional safety data required for licensing.
3. Labeling information: As specified under 21 CFR 201

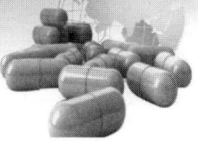

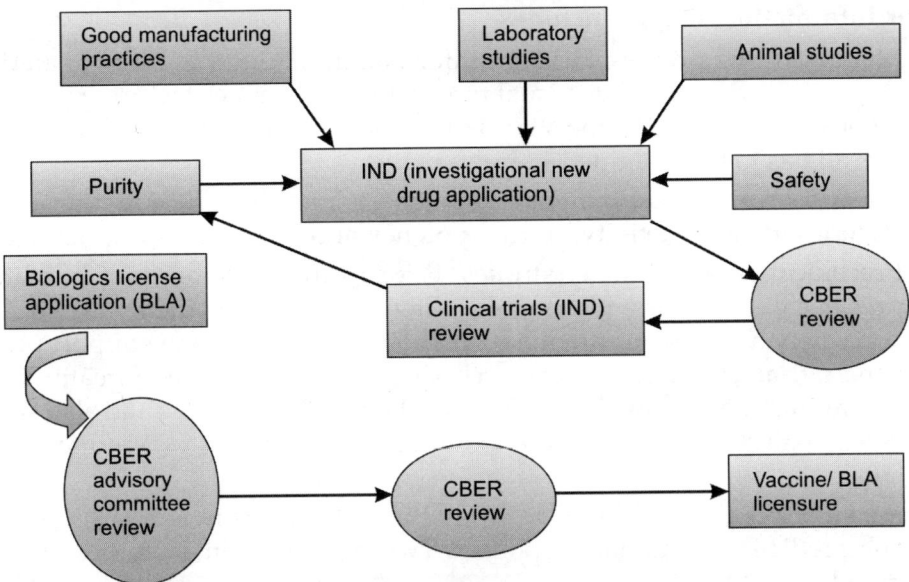

Fig. 2.5: Overview of BLA/vaccine approval process

Regulatory Approval Process of Vaccines

In order to gain approval for general medical use, the quality, safety and efficacy of any product must be demonstrated in Fig. 2.5. Demonstration of conformance to theses requirements particularly safety and efficacy, is largely attained by undertaking clinical trials. However, preliminary data especially safety data, must be obtained prior to drug's administration to human volunteers. Regulatory authority approval to commence clinical trials is based largely upon preclinical pharmacological and toxicological assessment of the potential drug in animals (Fig. 2.6).

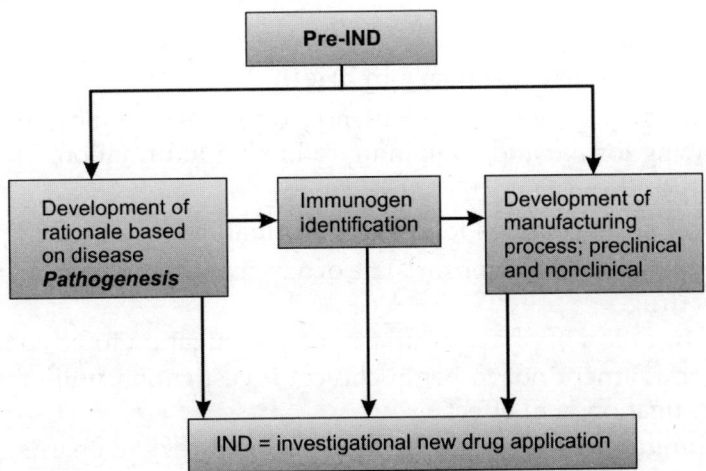

Fig. 2.6: Steps involved in pre-IND information

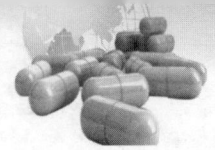

Major information sought includes

1. Manufacturing process: Here the information required is of raw material and reagents used, a complete visual representation of manufacturing flow should be provided indicating the steps in production, equipment and material used this all has to be submitted in brief.

2. Product characterization: Here key aspects on which information is sought includes identity, activity, purity, potency and stability of product.

3. Preclinical animal toxicity studies: Prior to the availability of human data, preclinical studies provide the sole source of data upon which activity [efficacy] and safety assessments are made. It should be adequate to support proposed clinical trial like, range of doses, schedule and/or duration of treatment, route of administration should mimic those planned for the clinic and also sufficient safety data should be available to determine end points for monitoring in the clinic.

The goal of pre-IND studies is to study the drug effects in animals, presumably enabling prediction of human responses. Two types of animal studies are usually performed:

• Toxicology studies, to explore safety of a drug.
• Pharmacokinetic studies, to explore exposure of a drug attained in animal experiments. This pharmacokinetic data is also used for interspecies scaling to predict human phase 1 doses.

Investigational New Drug Application for a Biologic Product

An Investigational New Drug (IND) Application is a request for authorization from the Food and Drug Administration (FDA) to administer an investigational drug or biological product to humans. Such authorization must be secured prior to interstate shipment and administration of any new drug or biological product that is not the subject of an approved New Drug Application or Biologics/Product License Application. This request is made by a sponsor (may be a pharmaceutical firm or an individual) to FDA.

IND content and format (summary in brief):

According to this act, a sponsor who intends to conduct a clinical trial has to submit IND in following format and containing following information:

1. Cover sheet (form FDA–1571) (roadmap)

   This cover sheet contains following information:

   i. Personal details of sponsor, date of application and name of investigational new drug.

   ii. Identification of phase or phases of investigation to be conducted.

   iii. A commitment not to begin clinical investigation until an IND covering investigation is in effect.

   iv. A commitment to setup IRB (institutional review boards) to continually review and approve studies.

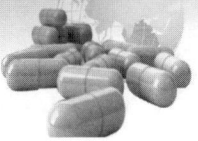

v. A commitment to conduct investigation in accordance to other applicable regulatory requirements.

vi. Personal details of person monitoring investigation.

vii. Personal details of person responsible under 21 CFR 312.32(1) (I) for review and evaluation of information relevant to safety of drugs.

viii. In case study is being conducted by CRO, then details of that CRO under 21 CFR 312.32(1) (VIII).

ix. Signature of sponsor under 21 CFR 312.32 (1) (IX).

2. A table of contents (what's where) under 21 CFR 312.32(2)

3. Introductory statement and general investigational plan (where you are headed) under 21 CFR 312.32 (3):

   i. Brief information about active ingredients of drug.

   ii. Summary of previous human experience with drug, if any.

   iii. Description of overall plan for investigation describing about rationale for study, indications to be studied and possible risks associated based on animal studies.

4. Investigator's brochure (preliminary package insert) under 21 CFR 312.32(5):

   Containing information about structure (if any), pharmacology, toxicology and safety profile of and anticipated risks and side effects of drug in accordance with ICH guidelines.

5. Protocols (plan for collecting safety and activity/efficacy data) under 21 CFR 312.32(6):

   For phase 1: provides an outline about general investigation plan with information like number of patients to be involved and dosing plan.

   For phase 2 and 3 detailed protocols are required with following information:

   i. A statement of objectives and purpose of study.

   ii. Details about investigators and institutional review board.

   iii. Criteria for patient selection and design of study.

   iv. Description about clinical procedures, laboratory tests or other measures to be taken to monitor effects of drug in humans.

6. Chemistry, manufacturing and control information (how you made the product and testing you did) under 21 CFR 312.32(7): This information needs to be submitted to assure proper quality, purity and strength of investigational drug. However, the type of information may vary depending upon the requirement of a particular phase of investigation and additional information appropriate to the expanded scope of investigation needs to be submitted when there is scaling up of production process.

7. Labeling information (for investigational use only).

8. Environmental analysis: All pre-marketing approvals of FDA regulated products are subject to the requirements of National Environmental Policy Act (NEPA) as defined by the council on environmental quality's regulations and as further described by FDA's NEPA implementing procedures. An

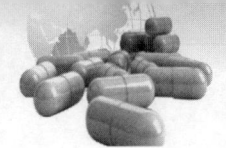

environmental impact statement is required if the manufacturer use, or disposal of the product is anticipated to cause significant environmental impacts [188].

Pharmacology and toxicological information (Data to conclude that it is reasonably safe to conduct clinical study) under 21 CFR 312.32(8): This requires appropriate pharmacological and toxicological information involving laboratory animals needs to be submitted on the basis of which sponsor has concluded that it is safe to conduct clinical studies.

Previous human experience with drug (same or different product) under 21 CFR 312.32(9): Under this section investigator is suppose to submit detailed information about previous human experience with investigational drug being marketed or investigated alone or in combination in US or any other region.

Additional information: Certain drugs like psychotropic drugs, radioactive drugs require additional information and incase material is submitted in any other information then complete english translation of that material is needed with 2 copies of each in addition to original copy and under 21 CFR 312.30 new protocol needs to be submitted whenever a sponsor intends to conducts clinical investigation with an exception from informed consent for emergency research.

IND Safety Reports

Safety of the subjects in all phases of trials is on the top of mind when FDA reviews any IND application. Therefore, major emphasis is always laid on maintaining IND through safety reports, annual reports to report any adverse events during the trials.

So in IND safety reports a sponsor must report in writing on FDA form 3500A any adverse experience associated with drug use that is both serious and unexpected or any findings from tests in laboratory animals that suggest a significant risk for human subjects including reports of mutagenecity or carcinogenicity within 15 days of receipt of such reports initially.

IND Annual Reports

A sponsor has to submit within 60 days of anniversary date that IND went into effect, a brief report of the progress of investigation including brief description of preclinical studies completed or in progress any significant phase 1 protocol amendment or information about drug's action like dose response, information from controlled trials, information about bioavailability and any significant manufacturing or microbiological changes made during the year.

Clinical Hold Policy

This is an order issued by FDA to sponsor to delay the proposed clinical investigation or to suspend an ongoing investigation.

Reasons for imposition of clinical hold:
1. Clinical hold of phase 1 study under IND
    i. If there is significant risk of human subjects of illness or injury.
    ii. Inadequate qualification of clinical investigators.

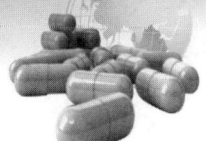

   iii. Investigator brochure is misleading, erroneous or materially incomplete.

   iv. IND does not contain sufficient information under 21 CFR 312.23 to assess the risk to subjects of proposed study.

2. Clinical hold of a phase 2 or phase 3 study under an IND

   i. Similar reasons as above.

   ii. Protocol or plan is clearly deficient in design to meet its objective.

Fast track, approval of biologics

Conditions for getting qualification under fast track drug development programme: According to Section 506 (a) (1) a drug in order be designated under fast track approval programme must be intended for:

a. A serious or life threatening condition. (The determination of seriousness of condition is a matter of judgment but is generally based on its impact on such factors as survival, day-to-day functioning, etc.)

b. Demonstrating the potential to address unmet medical needs (where in either the medical need is not addressed by existing therapy or there is no therapy for that medical need).

Review programs for fast track drug development: under the fast track drug development program, the sponsor may be considered for any of these benefits like:

1. *Priority review of BLA or marketing application*: Once the authorities are convinced that the drug under review is for some serious disease then the whole license process may be completed within 6 months.

2. *Submissions of portions of an application*: Under 506(c) FDA may consider portions of an application for review even before the complete BLA is submitted on a condition that sponsor will provide a schedule in which it will submit the necessary information to complete the application along with necessary fees under Section 736 of the act. This request must be submitted as an amendment to IND in triplicate along with form 1571 attached to it with clear identification of application designated as" request for submission of portions of an application".

3. *Accelerated approvals*: Applicants under fast track drug development programs may seek approval under accelerated approval regulations where in the application may be approved under Section 505(c) upon determination that product has an effect on the clinical end point or on a surrogate end point that is reasonably likely to predict clinical benefit. But approval under this section requires that sponsor conducts appropriate post approval studies to validate surrogate end points or otherwise confirm the effects of clinical end points. Also the sponsor has to submit the copies of all the promotional material related to fast track product at least 30 days prior to dissemination of the materials. But if the sponsor fails to conduct any

   a. Post-approval studies of fast track drug, or

   b. Post-approval study of the product fails to verify the clinical benefits of the product, or

c. Other evidences demonstrates that the given drug is not safe or effective under the conditions of use, or

d. The sponsor disseminates false or misleading promotional materials with respect to the products.

Then the authorities may withdraw the approval of a fast track product using expedited procedures.

Biological Drug Approval Process in the European Union

In the European Union (EU), biological medicinal product is an umbrella term covering a broad-spectrum of medicinal products, all of which are larger and more complex than chemically synthesized products. Biological medicines are defined as "product(s), the active substance of which is a biological substance".

EU GMP guidelines note that biologics "can be defined largely by reference to their method of manufacture". Examples of biological medicines include immunologic medicines; medicines derived from human blood and plasma; medicines developed by means of recombinant DNA technology, "controlled expression of genes coding for biologically active proteins in prokaryotes and eukaryotes including transformed mammalian cells", or hybridoma and mAb methods; and advanced therapy medicinal products.

The authority in charge of drug approval in the EU is EMEA. The committee that reviews drugs for human use (the CHMP, formerly CPMP) assesses the application, and then recommends whether a drug should have marketing authorization or not. There are 2 systems within the EMEA that pharmaceutical companies can use to license drugs. The first is the centralized system, the other is called the decentralized (or mutual recognition) system.

The centralized system

Any drugs for AIDS, cancer, neuro-degenerative conditions or diabetes have to be licensed this way. The process of application via the centralized system involves the pharmaceutical company filing an application with the EMEA. This is then passed to the CPMP. A preliminary review is undertaken early on in the process. The result is revealed to the company who may decide to continue with or withdraw the application. Representatives from two member states are selected to consider the application, one of which is chosen by the pharmaceutical company. These are called 'rapporteur' and 'co-rapporteur' member states. Their assessments form the basis for the final approval by the CPMP. The CPMP work to a strict time table laid down in EU law. An 'opinion' (positive or negative) has to be issued within 210 days of receipt of the application, although the company may stop the procedure at any time. If the opinion is negative the company must answer questions raised by the CPMP before the application can be progressed. If a positive opinion is issued, the EU Commission requests comments from other member states, which have 28 days to respond. Any objections to the rapporteur's decision are considered by the CPMP, which then makes a recommendation for or against an EU-wide licence. If a licence is recommended an European Public Assessment Report (EPAR) is produced and marketing authorization issued.

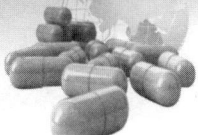

Decentralized (or mutual recognition) system

Under this system the CPMP coordinates the system, but does not take any part in the decision-making process unless there is disagreement between member states. After receipt of an application, the CPMP contracts one member state of the EU to assess the application. The contracted state is called the reference member state (RMS). The RMS is contracted to grant a licence within a maximum of 210 days. Once the RMS has approved the product other member states have 90 days to 'mutually recognize' the approval. The other countries may raise objections if there are concerns about safety, or major scientific or public health issues. However, some voices say that some countries object on purely political grounds. In this situation the CPMP acts as arbitrator and currently has 30 days to make a decision. The advice of the CPMP to the EU Commission is binding and each country then issues its own marketing authorizations.

Once a product has a marketing authorization it is then approved. The problem with this route is that it leads to different outcomes in different countries. Pharmaceutical companies believe that the mutual recognition procedure can, in some cases, offer a greater chance of approval as they simply avoid filing applications in member states where approval is doubtful. Historically, the UK licensing system has been one of the fastest in the world closely followed by the Swedish licensing system.

Accelerated approval or review

The EU system grants accelerated approval based on the seriousness of the disease, the absence or insufficiency of an appropriate alternative, and anticipation of high therapeutic benefit. Approval is often given on condition that actual clinical benefit is subsequently assessed. If a product has been assigned accelerated status, an opinion may be granted within 120 days of application. Following approval the company will be required to submit further data specifically requested by the licensing authority that may subsequently re-assess the application.

The Marketing Authorization Application—for Biologics: Contents and Approval Standard

Many biologics fall under the scope of the centralized marketing authorization procedure, which is mandatory for medicines developed through biotechnological methods (recombinant DNA technology; controlled expression of genes coding for biologically active proteins in prokaryotes and eukaryotes, including transformed mammalian cells; and hybridoma and mAb methods). For example, the following are subject to the centralized procedure: cell therapy, gene therapy, vaccines from strains developed through recombinant DNA technology (including gene deletion), and "any medicinal product for which a monoclonal antibody is used at any stage in the manufacturing process".

Nonetheless, some biologics are still approved at the member state level. For example, many vaccines do not fall within the scope of the centralized procedure. The EMA has published a guideline intended to harmonize the summaries of product characteristics and patient information leaflets for human vaccines.

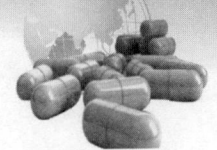

The approval standards for biotechnology products are the same as for chemically synthesized medicines. Both types of products must be safe and effective and have appropriate quality. Because of their special characteristics, however, biotechnology products must comply with several additional dossier requirements.

The MAA for a biotechnology product must meet the standard dossier submission requirements, as described in Article 8 of the Medicines Directive. Consequently, the MAA must generally comply with the CTD format, including with respect to:

  i. Module I (administrative information, including labeling and mock-ups),
 ii. Module 2 (various summaries),
iii. Module 3 (chemical, pharmaceutical, and biological information),
 iv. Module 4 (nonclinical reports), and
  v. Module 5 (clinical study reports).

MAAs for biologics also must meet special requirements. The applicant must thoroughly describe the manufacturing process:

1. Provide information on the origin and history of the starting materials;
2. Demonstrate that the active substance complies with specific measures for preventing the transmission of animal spongiform encephalopathies;
3. If cell banks are used, demonstrate that cell characteristics remain unchanged at the passage level for production (and beyond);
4. Provide information as to whether there are adventitious agents in seed materials, cell banks, pools of serum or plasma, and all other materials of biological origin, and, if it is not possible to avoid the presence of potentially pathogenic adventitious agents, show that further processing ensures elimination or inactivation of the agents;
5. If possible, base vaccine production on a seed lot system and established cell banks;
6. In case of medicines derived from human blood or plasma, describe the origin, criteria, and procedures for the collection, transportation, and storage of the starting material; and
7. Describe the manufacturing facilities and equipment. Other special rules apply certain types of biological medicines. For example, for plasma-derived medicinal products, the applicant must provide an information dossier, the Plasma Master File. MAAs for vaccines other than for influenza need to contain a Vaccine Antigen Master File. Special rules also apply to advanced therapy medicinal products, including gene therapies, somatic cell therapies, and tissue-engineered products.

Indian Regulatory System for Biologicals (Recombinant Products)

Regulation is a process by which governments ensure that the uncertainty and risks of a new technology can be contained within manageable limits. This is undertaken to overcome public resistance to technological advances and is incorporated into a receptive social context. Regulatory procedures devised to limit

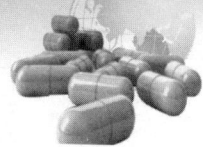

uncertainty, also to serve the purpose of channeling the flow of forthcoming public resistance and thus regulation, in fact, becomes an integral part of shaping of new technology.

Statutory bodies handling recombinant products

Rules notified under Environmental Protection Act (EPA), 1986 define the competitive authorities and composition of such authorities for handling all aspects of GMOs and products thereof. Presently there are 6 competent authorities:

The Recombinant DNA Advisory Committee (RDAC): This committee monitors from time to time the development in biotechnology at national and at international level. This committee prepared first rDNA guidelines in 1990, which were adopted by government for conducting research and handling GMOs in the country.

Institutional Biosafety Committee (IBSC): It is constituted by occupier or any person including R&D institutions handling GMOs and comprises head of institution, scientist doing rDNA work, medical expert and DBT nominee. Assists the occupier or any person including R&D institution prepare an emergency plan as per guidelines of RCGM (review committee on genetic manipulations).

Review Committee On Genetic Manipulation (RCGM): Under department of biotechnology has a function like:

1. To review all approved ongoing research projects involving high risk category and controlled field experiment research in areas namely human and animal health care, agriculture, industry and environmental management.

2. To visit site of experimental facilities periodically where projects with biohazard potential are being pursued and also at a time prior to the commencement of the activity to ensure that adequate safety measures are taken as per the guidelines.

3. To issue clearance for import/export of etiologic agents and vectors, germplasms, organelle, etc. needed for experimental work/training and research.

Genetic engineering approval committee (GEAC): This committee functions as a body under the Ministry of Environment and Forests and is responsible for approval of activities involving large scale use of hazardous microorganisms and recombinant products in research and industrial production from the environmental angle.

State Biotechnology coordination committee (SBCC): Formed in all states under chief secretary where research and applications of GMOs are contemplated. This committee coordinates the activities related to GMOs in the state with the central ministries. Besides it has powers to inspect, investigate and take punitive action in case of violations of statutory provisions through the appropriate state government departments.

District level committee (DLC): Constituted at the district level it is considered to be the smallest authorative unit to monitor the safety regulations in installations engaged in the use of GMOs in research and applications.

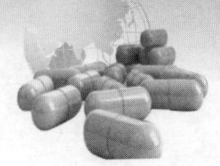

Regulatory requirements for recombinant products: Most of the recombinant products used as drugs are within the category of "new drugs" under Schedule Y of the Drugs and Cosmetics Act and Rules. For the production of recombinant products, there are certain regulatory mechanisms involved under the Environment (Protection) Act, 1986, and the Rules thereunder (1989) as they involve production of a GMO capable of manufacturing a particular product. Any company involved in the manufacture of recombinant product has to follow the EPA and the Rules thereunder before the production of a recombinant product as a drug.

General approval procedure for recombinant products:

1. A proposal is made before institutional biosafety committee (IBSC) and RCGM for granting approval.
2. Based on preclinical data review committee on genetic manipulation (RCGM) reviews it and conveys its recommendations to applicant, to Drugs Controller General of India (DCGI) and Genetic Engineering Approval Committee (GEAC).
3. The Recombinant DNA Advisory Committee (RDAC) approves the protocol and recommends for conducting clinical trials.
4. After completion of clinical trials IBSC examines the data from clinical trials and sends it to RCGM and DCGI for recommendation to GEAC for environmental release.

Where as for commercial release of recombinant products applicant must follow the provisions under Drugs and Cosmetics Act, because as per the drug and cosmetics (eight amendment) rules 1988 a substance of biological or biotechnological origin including vaccines (unless specified under Rule 21) and recombinant products shall be considered as new drugs; and as per the notification vide GSR No. 944(E) dated September 21, 1988, government has indicated the requirement of the activities for enabling the import or manufacture of biologicals.

Steps for getting approval for marketing and import of rDNA products in India:

i. Applicant makes request simultaneously in different formats to GEAC and to DCGI in 5 sets.
ii. Application is sent by GEAC and DCGI to various experts including department of biotechnology for their comments and recommendations.
iii. At this stage GEAC examines the application along with the comments and may ask for 21 sets of applications. In case the committee is not satisfied with the findings then it may ask applicant to further conduct clinical trials to clear any doubts therein with regards to safety and efficacy of the product.
iv. If the data is found satisfactory then GEAC may recommend to DCGI along with the condition to generate post-market surveillance information (phase 4 data). In case GEAC is not satisfied then it may direct applicant to apply afresh after generating the necessary clinical data under phase 3 clinical trial.
v. After getting approval from GEAC and also satisfying itself with the information therein DCGI may grant initial approval.

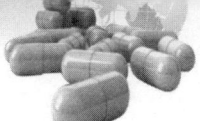

vi. Applicant then applies for form 10 along initial approval.

vii. Authorization for imports is granted to an applicant after it satisfies conditions as laid down by DCGI and GEAC.

viii. Marketing under EPA can be for a period of 2 to 4 years and can be reviewed after receiving an application after gong through post-market surveillance data.

Data required to be submitted with application for permission to market a new drug

i. Introduction: A brief description of the drug and therapeutic class to which it belongs.

ii. Chemical and pharmaceutical information: Includes information on chemical name, structure, specifications of ingredients including assay methods and stability data.

iii. Animal pharmacology: Includes information on pharmacological actions and pharmacokinetics.

iv. Animal toxicology information: Includes acute, long-term and local toxicity.

v. Human/clinical pharmacology (phase 1).

vi. Exploratory clinical trials (phase 2).

vii. Confirmatory trials (phase 3).

viii. Special studies: Includes bioavailability and dissolution studies.

Regulatory status in other countries: to include information about countries wherein drug is being marketed, approved under trial or has been withdrawn for any reason.

Marketing information: includes information on proposed monographs, drafts of labels and cartons, sample of pure drug substance with testing protocol.

Guidelines for generating preclinical and clinical data for rDNA vaccines and clinical data for rDNA vaccines, diagnostics and other biologicals

Biotechnology is poised for economic and social progress in the developed and developing countries. The biotechnology research, development and applications are growing at a rapid rate. This would lead to products and processes especially in pharmaceutical and health care sectors. Products and processes developed through recombinant DNA technology are already available in markets of developed and other countries. More and more products will be available in near future. So regulatory standards for recombinant DNA products are essential (Fig. 2.7). These guidelines specifically focus on safety, purity, potency and effectiveness of the product.

GOI : Government of India

DBT : Department of biotechnology

RDAC : Recombinant DNA advisory committee

IBSC : Institutional biosafety committee

RCGM : Review committee on genetic manipulation

DOEn : Department of environment

GEAC : Genetic engineering approval committee

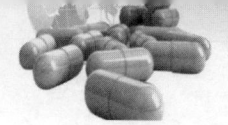

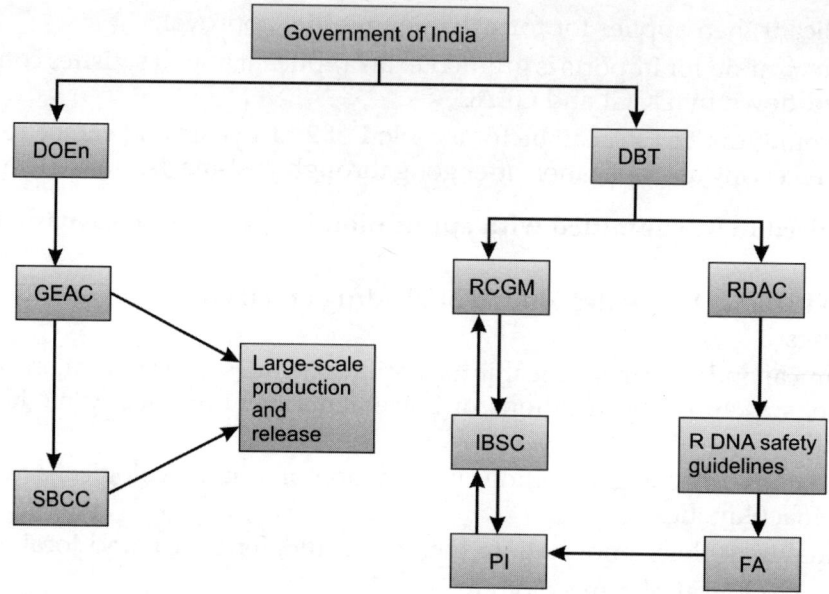

Fig. 2.7: Institutional mechanism for implementation of guideline framework

SBCC : State biotechnology coordination committee
PI : Principal investigator
FA : Funding agency

Specification and characterization information on rDNA vaccines and biological products.

Description in detail of the method of rDNA products includes:

  i. Host cells
  ii. Gene vector
 iii. All intermediate cloning procedures

Description of the method of sequence verification (such as restriction enzyme mapping, PCR, etc.)

1. Identity description
2. Description on recombinant products
3. Primary structure (amino acid sequences)
4. Secondary structure (disulphide linkages).

Monoclonal antibodies:

Identity by rigorous immunological/physiochemical characterization.

Potency (for recombinant vaccines and biologicals):

1. Production of specific recombinant reagents in transfected cell line.
2. Immune responses in mice
3. Hypersensitivity (guinea pig maximization test)
4. Permissible limits of potency.

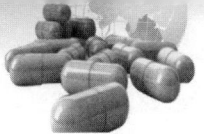

General safety test: To be performed in mice and guinea pigs on each lot of rDNA vaccines/biological to detect extraneous toxic contaminants potentially introduced during production.

Data on sterility tests as per Indian pharmacopoeia:

  i. Limits of purity.
 ii. Characterization of minor impurities like RNA, protein.
iii. Permissible limits of moisture, if lyophilized.
 iv. Pyrogenecity.
     Description of constituent materials like preservatives, etc.

Data on stability of finished formulation as per Indian pharmacopoeia guidelines.

Preclinical testing:

  i. General principles: The main objectives of these studies are to define physiological, toxicological and efficacious potential of rDNA products prior to initiation of human studies. Conventional approaches in preclinical tests of non-rDNA products may not be appropriate because of unique and diverse structural and biological properties of rDNA products.

 ii. Biological activity: It is evaluated using *in vitro* assays to determine the effects of product which are related to clinical activity. Cell line or cell cultures are used for this. These studies are used to determine receptor occupancy, receptor affinity and/or pharmacological effects and in case of monoclonal antibodies the immunological properties of the antibody should be described in detail including its antigenic specificity, affinity etc.

iii. Animal species selection: In normal circumstances for safety evaluation programs two relevant species should be used. All pharmacological, toxicological and immunological studies may be carried on one animal and efficacy studies on another in case no relevant species exists transgenic animals may be used.

 iv. Number/gender of animals: The sample size has direct bearing on ability to detect the toxicity and as far as possible both genders should be used for study.

  v. Dose selection and administration: The route and frequency should be decided after taking into account pharmacokinetic and bioavailability of the product.

 vi. Immunogenecity: For recombinant vaccines preclinical assessment must include immunological potency of the vaccine. The results would be required to choose a dose for clinical use. This study is also designed to collect information regarding the duration of antigen expression and whether long-term expression will result in tolerance or autoimmunity.

Specific considerations in preclinical testing:

  i. Safety pharmacology: Investigates undesirable pharmacological activity inappropriate animal model. The aim of this study is to establish functional effects on major physiological systems where in investigations may include use of isolated organ systems and not involving the whole organism.

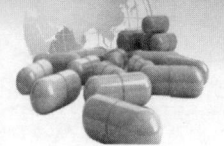
ii. Toxicology and pharmacokinetics: Aim here is to establish uniform guidelines for ADME (absorption, distribution, metabolism, excretion) studies for rDNA products. Since most of the recombinant substances are relatively large protein molecules, there are several characteristics that must be considered in their pharmacological and toxicological evaluation like poor oral absorption due to large molecular weight, protein/peptide proteolysis in blood or GI tract resulting in brief half life, often antigenic and often having reduced therapeutic effectiveness due to antibody neutralization.

iii. Immunotoxicity: The chief aspect of this evaluation is to assess the potential immunogenecity and hypersensitivity.

iv. Reproductive performance and developmental toxicity: Here rDNA vaccines/ biological should be evaluated for migration to gonadal tissue and possible germ line alternations in both male and female animals along with the scientific basis for conducting such an assessment.

Carcinogenicity studies: It is done to assess the carcinogenic potential of recombinant product.

Clinical trials (**note:** Clinical trials are performed as per requirements and guidelines in Schedule Y of Drugs and Cosmetics Act).

1. Human/clinical pharmacology (phase 1): In this case the potential of rDNA vaccine to produce immunogenic response should be monitored.

2. Exploratory clinical trials (phase 2): Where in the preventive/therapeutic potential of rDNA vaccine should be evaluated in normal subjects/patients. The minimum preventive/therapeutic dose of rDNA vaccine vis-à-vis immune responses should be determined.

3. Confirmatory trials(phase 3):

    i. For newer vaccines: The multicentric trial in large number of subjects/ patients as per regulatory requirement should be undertaken. The preventive or therapeutic efficacy of rDNA vaccine based on efficacy data of phase 2 clinical trial should be planned. The immunological parameters should be monitored in some cases at each center to generate data on ethnic, socioeconomic and cultural variations.

    ii. For established vaccines: For these vaccines a faster clearance method may be adopted. The data on abnormal/side effects should be considered including the outline of the method of manufacturing, construction of cell lines, etc. The data on post-market survey should also be provided.

In India all new drugs to be imported or to be produced locally for marketing authorization requires the permission of DCGI. DCGI may approve the import or local manufacture, provided he is satisfied with the information provided by applicant on the clinical trials data.

REGULATORY STRATEGIES FOR WORLDWIDE MARKETING OF BIOLOGICAL PRODUCTS

United States the FDA has adopted two regulations governing its acceptance of foreign clinical data, one applicable to supportive data and one applicable to data

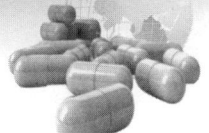

that form the sole basis for approval. Both regulations require the sponsor to meet certain conditions before the FDA will agree to use of the data.

First, the FDA accepts "well-designed and well-conducted" foreign, non-IND studies as "support" for an IND or BLA if two conditions are met. The FDA generally must be able to conduct an onsite inspection of the data, if necessary. The sponsor also must have conducted the study using GCP, as defined in 21 CFR § 312.120. For purposes of that regulation, GCP means standards that ensure the credibility of the results and the protection of subjects, including independent ethics board approval and documentation of subjects' informed consent. Complying with ICH E6, the GCP guidance, is one way—but not the only way—to meet this requirement. The FDA recently issued guidance on submitting information to demonstrate compliance with 21 CFR § 312.120. After these threshold criteria are met, the FDA will use the factors described in ICH E5, ethnic factors in the acceptability of foreign clinical data, to determine the scientific relevance of the data with respect to the US population and the need for additional bridging data to confirm their value.

Second, when foreign data are intended to form the sole basis for United States marketing approval, the sponsor must comply with GCP and meet three other criteria. The FDA must deem the foreign data to be "applicable to the US population and the US medical practice" using the criteria described in ICH E5. The clinical investigators must have "recognized competence." Finally, the data must be considered valid without the need for an onsite FDA inspection, or the FDA must be able to validate the data through such an inspection.

Foreign and Multinational Clinical Studies: Addressing Ethnic Factors

ICH E5 describes strategies to extrapolate clinical data generated in one region to support approval in another based on an assessment of ethnic factors' impact on the medicine's safety and efficacy. "Ethnic factors" include intrinsic factors, such as genetics and age, and extrinsic factors, such as regional clinical trial conduct and medical practice.

For the ICH E5 framework to apply, the clinical trial must meet the regulatory requirements (e.g. choice of control, trial endpoints, and key design features) of the region where approval is sought. Regulators then assess the medicine's sensitivity to ethnic factors using information about its PK and PD and their relationship to safety and efficacy. Based on the level of ethnic sensitivity, regulators will then determine whether existing data show the trials' relevance to the new region or whether a bridging study is necessary to confirm their relevance. For example, when the medicine is ethnically insensitive and extrinsic factors in the two regions are similar, regulators might not require a bridging study. Generally, one bridging study will suffice for extrapolation under ICH E5 unless the bridging study is too small to assess safety or does not confirm the relevance of the foreign data to the new region's population. In these cases, regulators in the new region likely will require additional data. Depending on the circumstances, a bridging study might use pharmacologic endpoints or might constitute a controlled clinical trial. Separate safety data might be needed when the sponsor does not need to perform a bridging efficacy study or when the efficacy study is not powered for safety.

ICH E5 and its companion Q&A guidance also discuss strategies for a multi-national trial to support simultaneous registration applications in multiple countries. The trial's goals would be to show efficacy in each region and to compare regional results to show insensitivity to ethnic factors. In designing these types of studies, sponsors should choose a primary endpoint that is acceptable to all regional regulatory authorities (or when this is impossible, collect data on all primary endpoints in all regions for comparison).

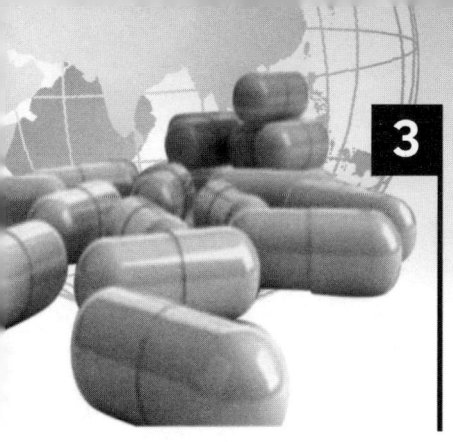

3

Regulatory Requirements for Product Approvals

OVER-THE-COUNTER DRUGS

Over-the-counter (OTC) drug is a category of pharmaceutical products which FDA defines an article intended for use in the diagnosis, cure, mitigation, treatment, or prevention of disease. Over-the-counter (OTC) pharmaceuticals are medicines that are available to the consumer for purchase without a prescription from a physician. This in itself is a broad definition and the scope of OTC pharmaceuticals varies as per different legal definitions that are adopted by various countries.

Whereas the US, Netherlands and Portugal all have only one class of OTC pharmaceuticals, UK has a two-tier system. In some European countries, there is another class of drugs called semi-ethical drugs that are sold over the counter, but like prescription drugs, are reimbursable from the national health care insurance provider or the government. Semi-ethical drugs contribute significantly to the OTC market of Germany, France, Belgium, Italy and Spain.

An OTC drug always contains at least one active pharmaceutical ingredient (API), intended to relieve the consumer's symptoms. These drugs are subject to slightly more stringent safety and efficacy standards than prescription drugs because consumers must be able to self-diagnose, self-treat and self-manage. They must be safe enough for consumers to use without the supervision of a doctor.

OTCs are used to treat a variety of health problems, including headaches, coughs and colds, fever, heartburn, etc. An OTC drug should not be confused with a dietary supplement (vitamins, minerals, etc.), which is regulated differently by the FDA.

APPROVAL PROCESS OF OTC DRUGS IN THE UNITED STATES

Introduction

Over-the-counter (OTC) drugs play an increasingly vital role in America's health care system. OTC drug products are those drugs that are available to consumers without a prescription. There are more than 80 therapeutic categories of OTC drugs, ranging from acne drug products to weight control drug products. As with prescription drugs, CDER oversees OTC drugs to ensure that they are properly labeled and that their benefits outweigh their risks.

OTC drugs generally have these characteristics:

i. Their benefits outweigh their risks

ii. The potential for misuse and abuse is low

iii. Consumer can use them for self-diagnosed conditions

iv. They can be adequately labeled

v. Health practitioners are not needed for the safe and effective use of the product

Office of Nonprescription Products

Two regulatory mechanisms exist for the legal marketing of OTC drug products:

1. NDA (regulations described in 21 CFR Part 314)

2. OTC drug monograph (regulations described in 21 CFR Part 330)

OTC drug products marketed under either mechanism must meet established standards for safety and effectiveness. Although we assess compliance with these standards differently under the two mechanisms, neither mechanism establishes higher standards for safety or effectiveness than the other. Under both mechanisms, products must be manufactured according to current good manufacturing practices (cGMPs) as defined in 21 CFR Part 210 and must comply with the labeling content and format requirements in 21 CFR Part 201 Subpart C.

New Drug Application

Legal marketing is under the authority of New Drug Application (NDA) or an Abbreviated New Drug Application (ANDA). An OTC drug product with active ingredient(s), dosage form, dosage strength, or route of administration new to the OTC marketplace is regulated under the NDA process. For example, a drug product previously available only by prescription (Rx) can be marketed OTC under an approved "Rx-to-OTC switch" NDA.

FDA must approve the NDA for an OTC drug product before that product can be marketed OTC. A drug manufacturer submits data in an NDA demonstrating a drug product is safe and effective for use by consumers without the assistance of a health care professional. FDA must review the data within an established timeframe, and the data submitted in an NDA remains confidential.

The drug manufacturer can only market the product with the specific formulation and exact labeling approved by FDA. To make a change, the manufacturer must submit an NDA supplement and FDA must approve that supplement.

A 505(b)(1) application, a 505(b)(2) application, or an abbreviated new drug application can be submitted.

OTC Drug Monograph

Legal marketing is in compliance with an OTC drug monograph. Unlike NDAs, which are based on drug **products**, monographs specify the **active ingredients** that can be contained within OTC drug products. An OTC drug product containing ingredients that comply with standards established in an applicable monograph is considered to be *"generally recognized as safe and effective" (GRASE)* and does not require specific

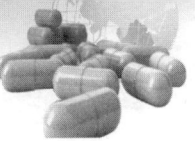

FDA approval before marketing. For example, OTC sunscreen drug products can be legally marketed if they contain ingredients, which comply with the standards established in the OTC sunscreen monograph for formulation, labeling, and testing. These products are listed in the United States Pharmacopoeia and are molecules that have been on the market for a long time. As they are classified as suitable for sale over the counter, they are deemed to be both efficacious and safe. The US FDA does not require manufacturers of these products to seek prior FDA approval in the form of a marketing authorization. However, manufacturing requirements to cGMP are still required with the data being made available upon request by the FDA. The labeling claims of the product are to be as those laid out within the monograph (Table 3.1).

The assembly of data from scale-up is classed as the pre-registration phase by Bioprogress. However, the data does not need to be submitted but has to be available for inspection prior to launch. This shortens the regulatory pathway significantly. Required conditions for monographs:

1. Active ingredients
2. Dosage forms
3. Dose or concentration
4. Required labeling
5. Packaging and/or testing requirements (in some cases).

Monograph Establishment

Based on the advisory review different categories are defined

Category I: Generally regarded as safe and effective (GRASE)

Category II: Non-GRASE

Category III: Cannot determine if safe and effective; more data needed.

S.No.	OTC monograph	New drug application (NDA)
		Table: 3.1 Comparison of OTC and NDA drugs
1.	No pre-market approval required	Pre-market approval of NDA
2.	No filing fees	May require user fee if new clinical studies required
3.	Public process	Confidential filing
4.	Covers active ingredients/therapeutic classes	Drug product-specific
5.	No mandated FDA review timelines	Mandated FDA review timelines
6.	No marketing exclusivity	Potential marketing exclusivity if new clinical studies required
7.	FDA approval of brand name not required	FDA approval of brand name required

Contd.

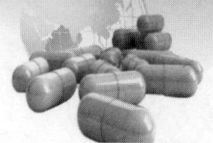

S.No.	OTC monograph	New drug application (NDA)
	Table: 3.1 Comparison of OTC and NDA drugs (Contd.)	
8.	No FDA approval required for post-marketing changes that conform to monograph	FDA pre-approval required for moderate or major changes FDA notification required for minor changes
9.	Clinical studies required for claims support only	May require to support: Safety and efficacy label comprehension
10.	Label must conform to monograph and "drug facts" label requirements	Label must conform to "drug facts" label requirements. Content of labelling to be developed and approved by the FDA based on the results of: • Clinical studies • Label comprehension studies • Self-selection studies • Actual use studies

Prescription to OTC Switch

Prescription to OTC switch refers to over the counter marketing of a product that was once a prescription drug product for the same indication, strength, and dose, duration of use, dosage form, population, and route of administration.

The prescription to OTC switch accomplished by following mechanisms, an efficacy supplement should be submitted to an approved NDA for a prescription product if the sponsor plans to switch the drug product covered under the NDA to OTC marketing status in its entirety without a change in the previously approved dosage form or route of administration. An NDA 505(b)(1) should be submitted if the sponsor is proposing to convert some but not all of the approved prescription indications to OTC marketing status.

An original NDA (505)(b)(1) or 505(b)(2) needs to be submitted if the sponsor plans to market either a new product OTC whose active substance, indication, or dosage form has never previously been marketed as OTC.

Data Submitted to the Agency

Data regarding OTC drug monographs can be submitted by anyone- such as a drug company, health professional, consumer, or citizen's group. If the submission is a request to change an existing OTC drug monograph or is an opinion regarding an OTC drug monograph, it needs to be submitted in the form of a citizen petition or as correspondence to an established monograph docket. However, if no OTC drug monograph exists, data must be submitted in the format as outlined in the code of federal regulations (CFR) Section 10.30.

Data is submitted to the dockets management branch where it is logged in and a copy is made for the public files. The data is then forwarded to the Division of Over-the-Counter Drug Products for review and action.

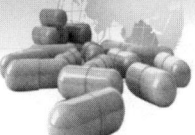

Review by CDER

When the submission is received in the Division of OTC Drug Products, a project manager conducts an initial review to determine the type of drug being referenced and then forwards the submission to the appropriate team for a more detailed review. The team leader determines if the submission will need to be reviewed by other discipline areas in the review divisions, such as chemists or statisticians, or by other consultants, such as those from other centers or agency offices. The submission is then forwarded to a team member for review.

If the submission is a comment or opinion on a specific rule or OTC drug monograph, there is no deadline established for CDER to respond. However, if the submission is a petition or request to amend a monograph, or request to have a drug approved based on an existing monograph, the OTC division has 180 days to review the data and respond to the submitter.

When the submission is reviewed, the drug is categorized through the monograph rulemaking process as follows:

1. Category I—generally recognized as safe and effective and not misbranded.
2. Category II—not generally recognized as safe and effective or is misbranded.
3. Category III—insufficient data available to permit classification. This category allows a manufacturer an opportunity to show that the ingredients in a product are safe and effective, or, if they are not, to reformulate or appropriately re-label the product.

CDER also oversees OTC drug labeling because the safety and effectiveness of OTC drug products depend not only on the ingredients but also on clear and truthful labeling that can be understood by consumers.

When the initial review is complete and other consult requests have been received, a "feedback letter" outlining CDER's recommendations may be prepared for the submitter. The recommendations will vary depending on the type of data submitted. For example, a response based on a request to amend a monograph may contain explanations approving or disapproving the amendment. If the submitter is not satisfied with the recommendations made by the division, the submitter may request a meeting to discuss any concerns.

OTC Advisory Committee Meeting

Advisory committee meetings are usually held to discuss specific safety or efficacy concerns, or the appropriateness of a switch from prescription to OTC marketing status for a product. Usually the OTC advisory committee meets jointly with the advisory committee having specific expertise in the use of the product.

APPROVAL PROCESSES OF OTC PHARMACEUTICALS IN EUROPE

Introduction

OTC products are called "non-prescription medicines" in the EU. The market authorization process for these products is similar to that of drugs, with the same marketing authorization form required. Section 2.3 of the marketing authorization application form asks for "legal status", and it must state on the box "not subject to medical prescription." All of the other requirements for OTC product registration are the same as those for prescription drugs.

Dual Regulatory Status in Europe

Dual regulatory status (DRS) is defined as having the same molecule and the same brand name simultaneously as in the Rx and the OTC markets. However, the Rx and the OTC drugs may have different strengths and/or indications. Prescription and OTC drugs can differ in strength, dosage, packaging, added indications, and so on. For example, for the sake of safety, the dosage of OTC drugs can be lower than that of prescription drugs. The dosage form can be altered to have a product that dissolves faster. The packaging can be attractive or consumer-friendly. However, at the same time, the company has to conduct clinical trials for stability, formulations and packaging criteria.

DRS are fairly common in certain markets, particularly the European markets like the UK and Germany. However, it is not widely practiced by ethical drug manufacturers in the US. It has a number of advantages over a simple Rx-to-OTC switch and as a result has become an important part of prescription drug manufacturer's strategies. The benefits offered by DRS can be summarized as follows:

1. Pharmaceutical companies apply for a dual status just before patent expiry for a molecule. This can offer a continuation of patent protection for prescription products and also the OTC products for a period of three years by obtaining a Waxman-Hatch extension, while further trials are executed.

2. Companies can capitalize on the prescription brand image to ensure faster popularity of the OTC brand.

3. Lower dose OTC formulations would have a better safety margin, than their prescription counterparts. This would facilitate OTC approval of the manufacturer's application from the regulatory authorities.

4. Advertising regulations governing OTC products are more relaxed than for prescription drugs, particularly in Europe. Thus, the advertising promotions for OTC products can also motivate consumers to ask physicians to prescribe the same brand name Rx products.

Rx-to-OTC Switching

Introduction

Rx-to-OTC switching increases the number of drugs available OTC and ensures that the drugs are available for self-medication, without the prescription from a physician or a pharmacists supervision. Rx-to-OTC switching has been the dominant factor in the growth of the OTC market in recent years.

In the past, switches in therapeutic categories, including analgesics, respiratory, feminine products, gastrointestinal and smoking cessation areas have fuelled growth in the OTC market. New drugs with specific pharmacological actions, such as

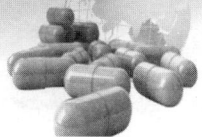

histamine H2-receptor antagonists, NSAIDs and nicotine preparations for smoking cessation have been successfully reclassified from prescription to non-prescription status in many countries.

Differences in Switching Policy Across Countries

In the process of switching a drug from prescription to non-prescription status, the responsibility for the change of legal status lies exclusively with the regulatory authority of that particular country. Hence, there are considerable differences between countries as certain drugs, which may be available as OTC pharmaceuticals in one country, may be available only on prescription in a different country (Table 3.2).

The UK has one of the most liberalized environments for Rx-to-OTC switches. This is because the government taxation finances the NHS, which provides health care to the majority of the citizens. The NHS bears the cost of the medication prescribed by a physician and hence the government recognizes self-medication as a viable form of cost containment. In the US, the approval procedure for Rx-to-OTC switches is significantly more stringent, because any drug approved for OTC sale would be available across any retail outlet and not just within pharmacies. The FDA does not recognize a third class of semi-ethical drugs and is very cautious when considering a new drug or indication for switch approval. Furthermore, the majority of health care in the US is provided by health care insurers such as Health Maintenance Organizations (HMOs) and not by the government. Thus, the government, on its own, is not inclined to reform the laws, which govern OTC drug classification for health care cost containment.

Table 3.2: Comparative status of drugs (Rx, OTC) in various countries							
Ingredient	*Japan*	*US*	*France*	*Germany*	*Italy*	*Spain*	*UK*
Ketoprofen	1994	1995	1997	1998	OTC	Rx	1993
Naproxen	Rx	1994	Rx	Rx	1994	OTC	Rx
Clotrimazole (topical)	1980	1989	OTC	OTC	OTC	OTC	OTC
Clotrimazole (vaginal)	Rx	1990	OTC	1994	Rx	Rx	1992
Ketoconazole	Rx	1997	1998	1992	OTC	Rx	1995
Acyclovir (topical)	Rx	Rx	1997	1992	Rx	2000	1993
Minoxidil (topical)	1999	1996	1998	Rx	OTC	OTC	1994
Beclomethasone (nasal)	Rx	Rx	Rx	1997	Rx	Rx	1994
Cimetidine	1997	1995	1997	Rx	1993	1996	1994
Famotidine	1997	1995	1996	1999	Rx	1996	1994
Loperamide	1989	1988	OTC	1993	1998	1996	OTC
Ranitidine	1997	1995	1997	1999	Rx	1997	1994
Nicotine (gum)	Rx	1996	1996	1994	OTC	1995	1991

Note: The year corresponds to the Rx-to-OTC switch

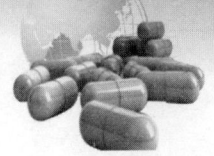

Drivers for Rx-to-OTC switching

Rx-to-OTC switching (Fig. 3.1) has been driven primarily by the commercial interests of pharmaceutical companies and by the desire of governments to curtail their national drug bills.

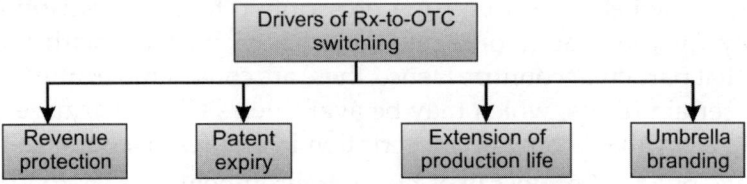

Fig. 3.1: Drivers of Rx-to-OTC switching

Revenue Protection

Pharmaceutical companies are in favor of Rx-to-OTC switching as an effective mechanism for profit protection. Pharmaceutical companies are increasing their basket of offerings for the self-medication market segment by shifting currently available prescription medicines to OTC status.

Patent expiry

A primary reason for switching a drug to OTC status is to maintain the revenue stream of the drug even after it has lost patent protection. Companies incur huge costs in the drug development process and, when the product patent expires, generic companies are likely to introduce cheaper versions of the same molecule and the discoverer is likely to lose market share, as some customers switch to the low cost generics. Moreover, in certain cases, when the product approaches maturity, companies have to adopt strategies to extend the product lifecycle and sustain revenues.

Growth in the OTC market has proved that creating new opportunities is not just a last resort, but also a feasible option for manufacturers to create new opportunities.

However, the successful switching of products from the Rx environment to the OTC market requires a vital understanding of these different markets, since success in the former does not necessarily guarantee success in the latter. For a prescription drug to become an OTC product, the following criteria need to be met:

i. The product should have been used extensively or in large volumes;

ii. It should have been marketed as a prescription product for at least five years.

iii. However, the period varies from country to country. No such timeframe is specified by the EU, while it is three years for New Zealand, six years for Japan, and up to 10 years for the Philippines;

iv. It should not have given any cause for concern during its adverse events and the frequency of such events should not have increased unduly during the marketing period.

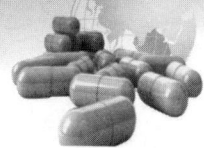

The reason for having a specified period is that the adverse events or the need for major changes in the product information are reported during the first three to five years after marketing, with the help of systems that effectively monitor drug safety.

Extension of product life

The entry of a more effective product or technology can also lead to a decline in the sales value of a prescription drug, which may also prompt a switch to OTC status as a possible treatment for less serious conditions. The FDA approved a new ethical treatment for ulcers in 1995, which could completely eradicate the disease. The new treatment, which combines the use of a proton pump inhibitor and an antibiotic, has replaced the older, H2-receptor antagonist therapies which are aimed at simply reducing stomach acidity. As a result, the older class of ethical drugs is becoming obsolete and companies have switched these drugs to OTC status in order to revive sales. H2-receptor antagonists have been switched for the less serious condition of heartburn and dyspepsia caused by excess acid in the stomach and they include brands such as Pepcid AC (famotidine), manufactured by J&J, Merck Consumer Pharmaceuticals.

Umbrella branding

Umbrella branding refers to the process of launching an OTC brand with the same brand name for a drug that was previously available through prescription only. This is also a driver for Rx-to-OTC switches where some drugs are switched to OTC status in order to complement a company's existing product portfolio. The addition of a clinically proven substance to an OTC portfolio can reinforce the image of the existing range and can add credibility in the market. This can have a synergistic effect on sales for both the existing range and the switched product. It also provides an opportunity to create a platform for developing line extensions around the original brand as well as allowing penetration in other segments of the OTC market.

REGULATORY REQUIREMENTS FOR PRODUCT APPROVALS: MEDICAL DEVICE

Definition of Medical Device

A "medical device" is broad term and includes wide range of equipment, consumable and disposable items used in diagnostic imaging, clinical laboratory, critical and routine patient care, patient monitoring and surgical procedures (Fig. 3.2). It also includes equipment used for assistance in cardiovascular, orthopedic, respiratory, ophthalmic, auditory, neurology, urinary, etc. disorders and self care equipment.

The definition of a medical device appears in Section 201(h) of the US Federal Food, Drug, and Cosmetic Act. **A device is**: " ... *an instrument, apparatus, AM.*

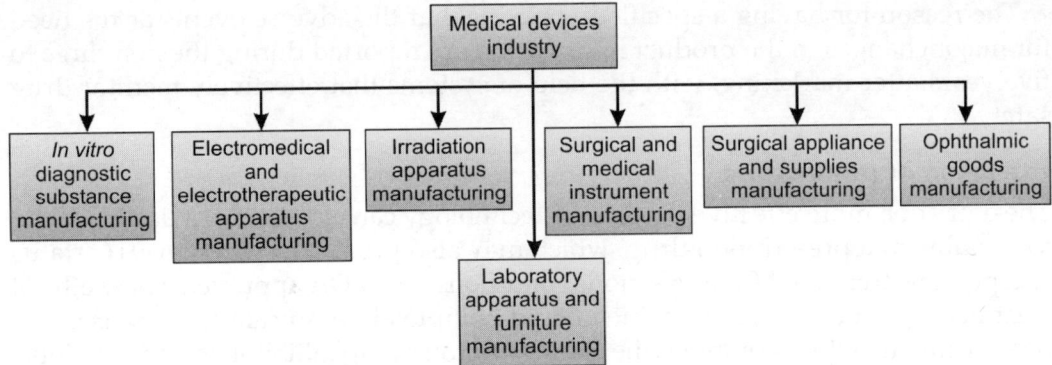

Fig. 3.2: Components of medical device industry

Medical device is implement, machine, contrivance, implant, *in vitro* reagent, or other similar or related article, including a component, part or accessory, which is:

a. Recognized in the official national formulary, or the United States Pharmacopoeia, or any supplement to them,

b. Intended for use in the diagnosis of disease or other conditions, or in the cure, mitigation, treatment, or prevention of disease, in man or other animals, or - intended to affect the structure or any function of the body of man or other animals, which does not achieve any of its primary intended purposes through chemical action within or on the body of man or other animals and which is not dependent upon being metabolized for the achievement of any of its intended purposes.

Approvals for Medical Devices in the USA

One of the most difficult aspects of getting a medical device to market is *knowing where to begin, i.e.* what are the steps for marketing and in what order they are to be taken. Essentially, medical devices are subject to the general controls of the Federal Food, Drug & Cosmetic (FD&C) Act which are contained in the final procedural regulations in Title 21 Code of Federal Regulations Part 800–1200 (21 CFR Parts 800–1299). These controls are the baseline requirements that apply to all medical devices necessary for marketing, proper labeling and monitoring its performance once the device is on the market. It involves three steps to obtain marketing clearance from CDRH.

Step one (*Defining medical device*)

To market any product as medical device it should meet the definition of a medical device in Section 201(h) of the FD&C Act. For example, the product may be a drug or biological product that is regulated by a component in the FDA other than the Center for Devices and Radiological Health (CDRH) and for which there are different provisions in the FD&C Act or the product may be a medical device and is also an electronic radiation emitting product with additional requirements.

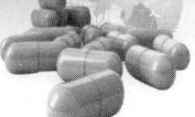

Step two (*Classifying the device*)

It is to determine how FDA may classify your device-which one of the three classes the device may fall into. Classification identifies the level of regulatory control that is necessary to assure the safety and effectiveness of a medical device. Most importantly, the classification of the device will identify, unless exempt, the marketing process (either premarket notification [510(k)] or premarket approval (PMA)) the manufacturer must complete in order to obtain FDA clearance/approval for marketing.

Step three (*Selecting the appropriate marketing application*)

It is the development of data and/or information necessary to submit a marketing application, and to obtain FDA clearance to market. For some submissions and most PMA applications, clinical performance data is required to obtain clearance to market. In these cases, conduct of the trial must be done in accord with FDA's Investigational Device Exemption (IDE) regulation, in addition to marketing clearance.

Other Requirements besides Marketing Clearance

It includes:
1. Premarket requirements: Labeling, registration, listing
2. Post-market requirements: Quality system, medical device reporting
3. Regulatory requirements
4. Documentation required

Premarket Requirements: Labeling, Registration, Listing

Before marketing clearance is obtained the manufacturer must assure that the device is properly labeled in accordance with FDA's labeling regulations. Once clearance for marketing is obtained, the manufacturer must register their establishment and list the type of device they plan to market with the FDA. This registration and listing process is accomplished by the submission of FDA Form 2891 and 2892.

Post-market Requirements: Quality System, Medical Device Reporting

Once on the market, there are post-market surveillance controls with which a manufacturer must comply. These requirements include the quality systems (QS) (also known as good manufacturing practices, GMPs) and medical device reporting (MDR) regulations. The QS regulation is a quality assurance requirement that covers the design, packaging, labeling and manufacturing of a medical device. The MDR regulation is an adverse event-reporting program.

In the US market, many medical devices are cleared for sale by a 510(k) pre-market approval. TÜV Rheinland of North America Inc. is accredited by the US Food and Drug Administration (US FDA) to carry out 510(k) reviews.

To sell the medical device in the US market, the Food and Drug Administration (FDA) will need a 510(k) submission for most Class II devices. With this submission the FDA can check whether the product is substantially equivalent to a product that is already approved in the United States and fulfils the US safety and effectiveness requirements.

   i. It will also be checked whether the product is suitable for an independent appraisal. This is the case for all products on the FDA's list of devices for third party review [106].

   ii. Than it will go ahead with the 510(k) documentation and send for assessment along with the documents to the FDA.

   iii. If a target date is agreed, it require less than four weeks for the review.

The FDA will then notify within 30 days at the latest of its decision on whether the 510(k) documents can be accepted.

Generally the notification is usually received within 14 days. The pre-market notification 510(k) is the most common method of approving a medical or IVD device in the USA.

Regulatory Requirements

With the exception of custom-made devices and medical devices manufactured in-house, medical devices pursuant to § 11, paragraph 1 MPG (Act on Medical Devices), as well as medical devices intended for clinical investigation, or *in vitro* diagnostic medical devices intended for performance evaluation, medical devices may only be placed on the market or put into service if they bear the CE marking.

   i. The CE marking shall be used.

   ii. For active implantable medical devices according to Annex 9 to Directive 90/385/EEC,

   iii. For *in vitro* diagnostic medical devices according to Annex X to Directive 98/79/EC,

   iv. For the other medical devices according to Annex XII to Directive 93/42/EEC.

The CE marking must be accompanied by the identification number of the relevant Notified Body which was involved in the conformity assessment procedure pursuant to Annexes 2, 4 and 5 to Directive 90/385/EEC, Annexes II, IV, V and VI to Directive 93/42/EEC, as well as Annexes III, IV, VI and VII to Directive 98/79/EC, which resulted in the right to affix the CE marking.

Documentation Required

The directive requires manufacturers to prepare for:

1. Class I devices

A declaration of conformity and technical documentation (article 11(5), annex VII section 3, Council Directive 93/42/EEC).

2. Custom made devices

A statement and documentation allowing an understanding of the design (Article 11(6), Annex VIII Council Directive 93/42/EEC) (Annex 6 Council Directive 90/385/EEC).

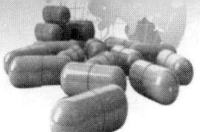

3. Devices covered by article 12

A declaration (Article 12 Council Directive 93/42/EEC)

There is no requirement to supply any of these documents when registering; however these may be inspected at any time by the Competent Authority for a period ending at least five years after the last product has been manufactured.

The Medical Devices Directive 93/42/EEC requires manufacturers or, their authorized representatives or others placing medical device(s) on the community market, to provide certain information to a Competent Authority in a Member State where they have a registered place of business.

MEDICAL DEVICES IN INDIA

Medical devices employed in internal or external use in the diagnosis, treatment, mitigation or prevention of disease or disorder in human beings or animals are considered to be "drugs" as notified by the central government in its official gazette after consultation with the Drugs Technical Advisory Board. Those medical devices not notified as drugs only require an import or manufacturing license and no quality check system exist for them.

Regulatory Framework

At the moment, in India there is no single comprehensive specific law regulating medical devices.

The import, manufacturing, sale and distribution of medical devices are regulated under the Drugs and Cosmetics Act, 1940 ("India Act"), the Drugs and Cosmetics Rules, 1945 ("Rules"); and the Central Drugs Standard Control Organization ("CDSCO"), under the Ministry of Health and Family Welfare ("Ministry") is the principal regulator.

A draft Bill on "Regulation of Medical Devices" ("the Bill") has been pending since 2006. Once implemented, it will, perhaps, streamline the medical devices sector. Until such time, one has to refer to multifarious regulations. With effect from March 1, 2006, the Ministry approved a set of procedures for the import as well as manufacture of medical devices in India.

The Drugs Technical Advisory Board, which provides technical guidance to CDSCO, proposed certain changes in the Rules, which among others provides a categorization of medical devices into four classes. This classification is based on the risk level, intended use and on adverse effect of the devices on the human body based on the potential risks associated with the technical design and manufacture of these devices. The classes of devices are:

1. Class A: Low risk devices and equipment such as thermometers and tongue depressors;
2. Class B: Low to moderate risk devices including hypodermic needles and suction equipment;
3. Class C: Moderate to high risk equipment like lung ventilators and bone fixation plates; and

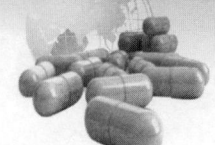
4. Class D: High risk devices such as heart valves and implantable defibrillators. The regulatory control becomes stringent with each progressive class and the conformity assessments are proportionate to device classification.

Import of Medical Devices

Presently, the import of medical devices is largely unregulated and medical devices can be freely imported into India. The purchaser (whether it is a government hospital, a private hospital or a doctor) evaluates the quality of the product being purchased.

Normally, the US Food and Drug Authority ("FDA") and the European Conformite Europeenne ("CE") approved products are preferred because of their better quality and performance.

It is necessary to follow the procedures for registering and obtaining a license as laid down under the Rules. Import licenses are conditional and granted for a period of three years.

Breach of any of the stipulated conditions may lead to the cancellation of the license.

1. To be registered in India, the imported device must be approved for sale in the manufacturer's country of origin. If the device has already received approval from an agency abroad, such as, the USFDA, evidence of such approval must be provided along with a copy of quality standard ISO/EN certification which assesses the quality and risk of the devices manufacturing facility.

2. Medical devices with prior approval from any of the recognized regulatory authorities, like FDA and CE are subjected to an abridged evaluation in India.

3. If a device is not approved for marketing in the country of origin, the importer has to submit additional evidence such as reports of clinical trials, details of sales, certificates of satisfactory use from medical specialists about the use of the device and details of product complaints, if any.

4. If a device incorporates a medicinal product, which is likely to act upon the body in conjunction with the device, it is pertinent to provide relevant data on the safety, quality, and usefulness of the medicinal substance used along with data on compatibility with medicinal products, clinical data and published articles, if any.

The manufacturer must also have complied with product standards and home country quality control requirements. The manufacturer of the devices, the importer or his agent must file an application to obtain a registration certificate with respect to the premises where the devices are manufactured and with regard to the devices. The product information and the undertakings with respect to product standards, safety and effectiveness requirements and quality systems in the country of origin are necessary to be furnished. Crucially, a brief description of the device, its intended use and method of use, medical specialty in which the device is used, the qualitative and quantitative particulars of the constituents, device master file with details of the manufacturing process/flow chart and the component/material used and risk

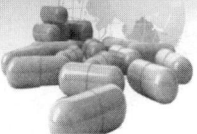

assessment as per ISO 14971 are necessary to be provided. Once a medical device reaches the market in India, the manufacturer has to adhere to requirements of post-marketing surveillance ("PMS") norms to systematically monitor the performance of the device. PMS involves procedures for maintenance of records, complaint handling, adverse incident reporting and procedures for product recall.

Manufacture of Medical Devices: It involves the following steps:

1. The manufacture of medical devices in India requires a license from the government.
2. An application for the license is made with a brief description of the manufacturing process, details of the manufacturing standards and "best practices" that will be followed by the company, as well as product evaluation, standards, and procedures for testing the device.
3. The Rules prescribed in Schedule M-III list mandatory "good manufacturing practices" that manufacturing companies must follow.
4. The law provides that any manufacturing can be done under the direction and supervision of only a whole-time employee of the manufacturer and who is qualified to do so.
5. India has several harsh industrial and labor laws that make the occupier of the manufacturing plant responsible for any violate in compliance.
6. The occupier is generally the managing director of the company that runs the manufacturing unit or a director on the board of directors and can be fined up to INR 0.2 million or imprisoned up to two years for any non-compliance.
7. As proposed under the bill, the regulatory authority sets up an expert committee to consider proposals and evaluate medical devices that do not have any benchmark certification. The committee after completing its assessment forwards its opinion regarding suitability of the device to the competent licensing authority which can grant permission for the device to be launched in the market.
8. The licensing authority after joint inspection and verification forwards the license to Central License Approving Authority (CLAA) for approval. The license is finally issued in form 28 of the Rules after due approval of CLAA. The stockist and retail sellers of medical devices are also required to obtain sales licenses from the respective state licensing authorities for medical devices.

Clinical Investigations

At present, clinical trial studies are not regulated in India. However, a set of good clinical practices guidelines laid down by the CDSCO govern clinical trials and specify the responsibilities, inter alia, of sponsors, investigators, and ethics committees.

1. In 2010, CDSCO released a guidance document on the requirements for conducting clinical trials of medical devices in India.
2. It is necessary to file an application with the CDSCO before conducting the study and the application should indicate the precise intent of the application.

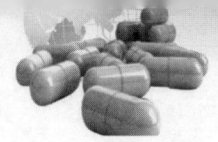

3. For safety and efficacy study, or a post-market study. The entity sponsoring the study must also submit a declaration on its letterhead prescribing the extent of delegation of responsibilities to an individual who is appointed as the principle investigator. It is also necessary to provide the global regulatory status of the device.

4. Global Harmonization Task Force ("GHTF") countries, i.e. the USA, Australia, Japan, Canada and the European Union are involved along with detailed technical data.

5. Though the document is still non-binding, it provides sufficient procedural information regarding the method to all stakeholders.

Medical devices: Quality standards

According to the guidance, all medical devices sold in this country should carry the Indian Conformity Assessment Certificate (ICAC) mark to indicate their conformity with the provisions of the schedule of the guidance to enable them to move freely within the country.

1. CLAA adopts and recognizes quality standard BIS 15575 or its revisions and quality standard ISO 13485 in respect of the specifications to be followed for quality for the manufacturer to demonstrate conformity with the relevant regulatory requirements. Any reference to the harmonized standards includes the monographs of the Indian pharmacopoeia and the US, the EU Pharmacopoeia wherever applicable, notably on surgical sutures and on combination of pharmaceutical and devices.

2. It is necessary that the labels on the packaging material for medical devices comply with the relevant ISO standards. It is also necessary to denote internationally accepted symbols regarding sterilization, single use, etc. as per ISO 15223-1:2007.

3. When medical devices are sold in bulk the packaging material of individual devices do not have to bear the date of manufacture, which must appear on the bulk packaging material.

4. Harsh regulatory standards are essential to ensure that the devices are tested, safe and with minimum adverse reactions. Standards regarding safety, risk elements, effectiveness, efficiency and performance of the medical devices need to be well established.

There are different proposals for regulating India's medical devices sector by different regulatory bodies, like amending the India Act and Rules proposed by the Ministry.

REGULATORY REQUIREMENTS FOR PRODUCT APPROVALS: HERBAL MEDICINES AND HOMEOPATHY

The objective of these guidelines is to propose to Member States a framework for facilitating the regulation of herbal medicines/products used in traditional medicine (TM). The proposed framework, which has a regional perspective, should help

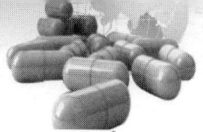

accelerate the establishment of appropriate mechanisms for registration and regulation of herbal medicines within SEAR, based on criteria for safety of use, therapeutic efficacy, quality control and pharmacovigilance. Traditional medicine involves not only the use of herbal medicines, but also use of animal parts and minerals. As herbal medicines are the most widely used of the three, and as the other types of materials involve other complex factors, this document will concentrate on herbal medicines.

Objectives

1. To classify the herbal medicines;
2. To propose regulatory requirements for the registration of each category of herbal medicines;
3. To set up minimum requirements for registration and regulation of herbal medicines.

Classification of Herbal Medicines

For practical purposes, herbal medicines can be classified into four categories, based on their origin, evolution and the forms of current usage. While these are not always mutually exclusive, these categories have sufficient distinguishing features for a constructive examination of the ways in which safety, efficacy and quality can be determined and improved.

Category 1: Indigenous herbal medicines

This category of herbal medicines is historically used in a local community or region and is very well known through long usage by the local population in terms of its composition, treatment and dosage. Detailed information on this category of TM, which also includes folk medicines, may or may not be available. It can be used freely by the local community or in the local region.

Category 2: Herbal medicines in systems

Medicines in this category have been used for a long time and are documented with their special theories and concepts, and accepted by the countries. For example, Ayurveda, Unani and Siddha would fall into this category of TM.

Category 3: Modified herbal medicines

These are herbal medicines as described above in categories 1 and 2, except that they have been modified in some way—either shape, or form including dose, dosage form, mode of administration, herbal medicinal ingredients, methods of preparation and medical indications. They have to meet the national regulatory requirements of safety and efficacy of herbal medicines.

Category 4: Imported products with a herbal medicine base

This category covers all imported herbal medicines including raw materials and products. Imported herbal medicines must be registered and marketed in the countries of origin. The safety and efficacy data have to be submitted to the national authority of the importing country and need to meet the requirements of safety and efficacy of regulation of herbal medicines in the recipient country.

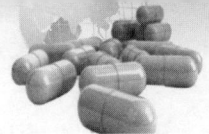

Minimum requirements for assessment of safety of herbal medicines

Safety category

A drug is defined as being safe if it causes no known or potential harm to users. There are three categories of safety that need to be considered, as these would dictate the nature of the safety requirements that would have to be ensured.

1. Category 1: safety established by use over long time
2. Category 2: safe under specific conditions of use (such herbal medicines should preferably be covered by well-established documentation)
3. Category 3: herbal medicines of uncertain safety (the safety data required for this class of drugs will be identical to that of any new substance)

Data will be required on the following:

1. Acute toxicity
2. Long-term toxicity

Data may also be necessary on the following:

1. Organ-targeted toxicity
2. Immunotoxicity
3. Embryo/fetal and prenatal toxicity
4. Mutagenicity/genotoxicity
5. Carcinogenicity

General considerations for assessment of safety of herbal medicines

Any assessment of herbal medicines must be based on unambiguous identification and characterization of the constituents. A literature search must be performed. This should include the general literature such as handbooks specific to the individual form of therapy, modern handbooks on phytotherapy, phytochemistry and pharmacognosy, articles published in scientific journals, official monographs such as WHO monographs, national monographs and other authoritative data related to herbal medicines and, if available, database searches in online or offline databases, e.g. WHO adverse drug reaction database, National Library of Medicine's Medline, etc. The searches should not only focus on the specific herbal medicinal preparation, but should be include different parts of the plant, related plant species and information originating from chemotaxonomy. Toxicological information on single ingredients should be assessed for its relevance to the herbal medicines.

Specific requirements for assessment of safety of four categories of herbal medicines

Before any category of herbal medicine listed above is introduced into the market, the relevant safety category needs to be reviewed and the required safety data obtained, based on that particular safety category.

Category 1: Indigenous herbal medicines

These can be used freely by the local community or region, and no safety data would be required. However, if the medicines in this category are introduced into

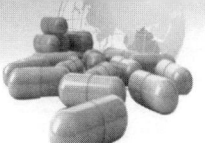

the market or moved beyond the local community or region, their safety has to be reviewed by the established national drug control agency.

If the medicines belong to safety category 1, safety data are not needed. If the medicines belong to safety category 2, they have to meet the usual requirements for safety of herbal medicines. Medicines belonging to safety category 3, i.e. 'herbal medicines of uncertain safety', will be identical to that of any new substance.

Category 2: Herbal medicines in systems

The medicines in this category have been used for a long time and have been officially documented. Review of the safety category is necessary. If the medicines are in safety categories 1 or 2, safety data would not be needed. If the medicines belong to safety category 3, they have to meet the requirements for safety of 'herbal medicines of uncertain safety'.

Category 3: Modified herbal medicines

The medicines in this category can be modified in any way including dose, dosage form, mode of administration, herbal medicinal ingredients, methods of preparation, or medical indications based on categories 1 and 2.

The medicines have to meet the requirements of safety of herbal medicines or requirements for the safety of 'herbal medicines of uncertain safety', depending on the modification.

Category 4: Imported/exported products with a herbal medicine base

Exported products shall require safety data, which have to meet the requirements for safety of herbal medicines or requirements for safety of 'herbal medicines of uncertain safety', depending on the safety requirement of the importing/recipient countries.

Disease

1. *Acute disease:* Diseases that have a rapid onset and a relatively short duration.
2. *Chronic disease:* Diseases that have a slow onset and last for long periods of time. Diseases of acute onset could also progress to a chronic state. In most cases, severe diseases refer to a life-threatening illness or those diseases in which delayed treatment will lead to deterioration of the disease state or loss of capability to cure them. For example, severe cardiovascular, gastrointestinal, endocrine, hematological diseases, and immune disorders and diseases fall into this group.
3. *Health condition:* Problems related to health conditions are those which, with time, could recover spontaneously, even without any medical intervention, e.g. loss of appetite, hay fever, menopause, etc. The efficacy for this category could be supported by data in existing well-established documents such as national pharmacopoeia and monographs as well as other authoritative documents such as WHO monographs. Preclinical and clinical data of efficacy may not be necessary (Tables 3.3 and 3.4).

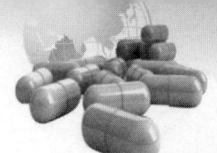

Table 3.3: Summary of the efficacy data requirements for the three types of disease and conditions

Type of disease	Preclinical data of efficacy	Clinical data of efficacy	Other data or information required
Acute	Needed	Control trial needed	
Chronic	May be needed	Clinical data may or may not be needed	
Health condition	May not be needed	May not be needed	Supported by well-established documents like pharmacopoeia and monographs

Table 3.4: Requirements data for the evaluation of efficacy of traditionally used herbal medicines with limited modifications

Traditionally used herbal medicines with well-established documentation	Preclinical data of efficacy	Clinical data of efficacy
No change based on traditional use	Not needed	May not be needed
Dose	May be needed	Needed
Dosage form	May be needed	Needed
Mode of administration	May or may not be needed	Needed
Medical indication	Needed	Needed
Changes in addition	Needed	Needed
Herbal deletion medicinal ingredients	May or may not be needed	May or may not be needed
New combination	Needed	Needed
Part of medicinal plant used	Needed	Needed
Methods of preparation	Needed	Needed

The following are terms related to the tables:

1. *Preclinical data:* These include efficacy of laboratory test and data regarding the standard dose and dosage form.
2. *Clinical data of efficacy:* This refers to 'clinical research' in WHO General Guidelines for Methodologies on research and evaluation of herbal medicines.
3. *Addition:* This means the addition of one or more plants or ingredients into traditionally used formulas.
4. *Deletion:* This refers to the deletion of one or more plants or ingredients from traditionally used formulas.
5. *New combination:* Two or more traditionally used formulas are put together.

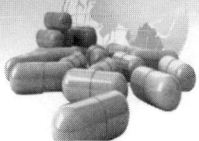

Minimum requirements for assessment of the efficacy of herbal medicines

1. The assessment of efficacy for herbal medicines in categories 1 and 2 are not required if they are used locally.
2. For medicines in category 3, preclinical data and clinical data may or may not be required depending on the modification(s), which are given in Table 3.4.
3. For medicines in category 4, efficacy data are required.

Quality Assurance of Herbal Medicinal Products

Quality assurance of herbal medicinal products is the shared responsibility of manufacturers and regulatory bodies. National drug regulatory authorities have to establish guidelines on all elements of quality assurance, evaluate dossiers and data submitted by the producers, and check post-marketing compliance of products with the specifications set out by the producers as well as compliance with good manufacturing practices (GMP).

The manufacturers have to adhere to good agricultural and collection practices (GACP), GMP and good laboratory practice (GLP) standards, establish appropriate specifications for their products, intermediates and starting materials and compile a well-structured, comprehensive documentation on pharmaceutical development and testing. The producers should make continued efforts to improve standards and adapt them to the present state of knowledge. A cooperative approach between different manufacturers, e.g. by establishing drug master-files for specifications and quality control, should be encouraged.

Coordinating Quality Control

A coordinating agency on GACP should be established to facilitate the availability of good-quality herbal medicines to the market by giving training and advice to small producers and farmers. To encourage implementation of GACP, incentives should be given to producers of botanical raw materials. These include giving technical and logistic support in the selection of appropriate sites for agricultural production, providing seeds and seedlings, selecting fertilizers and pesticides, providing or giving advice on machinery for harvesting and primary processing. The government should honour efforts by issuing certificates to producers and farmers who adhere to the GACP, based on the country situation. Implementation of such requirements is only possible if the production and marketing of herbal medicines is subject to an adequate registration scheme by a drug regulatory authority.

Quality assurance

Elements of quality assurance are:

1. Adherence to GACP, GMP and GLP guidelines;
2. Setting specifications; and
3. Quality control measures.

Quality control for herbal medicinal products

All herbal-based medicinal products should meet the requirements for safety, efficacy and quality, as per the Categories of Herbal Medicines.

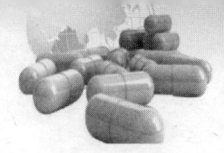

All imported herbal medicinal products need to meet the requirements for safety, efficacy and quality control regulations in the importing countries. To control the quality of imported herbal medicinal products, the following requirements should be taken into consideration.

Licensing authority

Licensing for importers, wholesalers, manufacturers and assemblers of herbal medicinal products should be issued by the national drug regulatory authority. Dealers of imported herbal medicinal products need to apply for one or more of the licenses depending on the type of business involved, such as license of importers, wholesalers, manufacturers and assemblers.

Import license

The responsibility of applying for an import license shall rest with local companies which are approved by the licensing authority to import herbal medicinal products and sell them in the importing countries.

The following information related to the importing company is required for the application of an import license:

1. Particulars of the company.
2. Particulars of the person making the application on behalf of the company.
3. Certificate of company/business registration.
4. Layout plan of the store.

Importers are required to provide information on each imported herbal medicinal product they deal with, and will be allowed to deal in approved products only. Detailed requirements for each imported herbal medicinal product are as follows:

1. Full product formula (in the languages of the importing and exporting countries)
2. A set containing labels, pamphlet, carton and specimen sales pack (in the languages of the importing and exporting countries, if necessary).
3. Particulars of manufacturer(s) and assembler(s).
4. Manufacturer's licence or certificate from the drug regulatory authority of the manufacturing country of origin.
5. Pre-export notification and certificate of free sale of the herbal medicinal product should be obtained from the concerned authority.

Based on the above mentioned minimum requirements, each national drug regulatory authority could develop its own requirements for quality control of imported herbal medicinal products.

Guidelines related to Good Agricultural and Collection Practices (GACP) and Good Manufacturing Practices (GMP)

The coordinating agency should adhere to the principles set out in the WHO Guidelines on good agricultural and collection practices for medicinal plants (for GACP) and manufacturers and assemblers should follow WHO good manufacturing

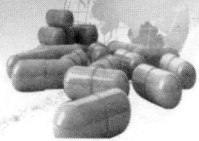

practices (for GMP). Manufacturers of herbal medicines should obtain a license and register their products. The quality control system for production should be in place. The implementation of a credible concept of quality assurance, e.g. identifying and eliminating potential sources of contamination, should be a primary goal of the manufacturers rather than the implementation of all individual technical aspects.

The following areas should be considered while studying the WHO guidelines:

1. Control of raw materials (refer to the GACP and quality control methods for medicinal plant products).
2. Control of starting materials and intermediate substances.
3. In-process control (standard operating procedure for processing methods should be mentioned).
4. Finished product control (it should be performed with reference to the control of raw materials, starting materials and intermediate substances).

Guidelines Related to Quality Control

The purpose of quality control is to ensure quality of the products by adhering to appropriate specifications and standards. Information on appropriate standards can be found in official pharmacopoeias, monographs, handbooks, etc. In choosing analytical methods, the availability, robustness and validity of the methods must be considered, such as microscopic identification, thin layer chromatography (TLC), titration of active substance and, if possible, a full validation of more sophisticated methods, such as high-performance liquid chromatography (HPLC), gas chromatography (GC), and gas chromatography-mass spectrometry (GC-MS). If such advanced methods are used, a full validation for each test would be necessary.

Product information for registration

This should include all necessary information on the proper use of the product. The detailed information of the herbal medicinal products should include the following requirements for registration:

1. Quantitative list of ingredients; if this is difficult, it could be replaced by including the plant names and plant parts used (i.e. Latin name).
2. Full product formula for imported herbal-based medicinal products (in the language of the importing and exporting countries).
3. A set containing labels, pamphlet, cartoon and specimen sales pack.
4. Particulars of manufacturer(s) and assembler(s).
5. Manufacturer's licence or certificate from the drug regulatory authority. Pre-export notification and certificate of free sale of the herbal-based medicinal product should be obtained from the concerned authority.
6. Brand name of product.
7. Dosage form.
8. Indications.
9. Dosage.

10. Mode of administration.
11. Duration of use.
12. Adverse effects.
13. Contraindications, warnings, precautions and major drug interactions, if possible.
14. Date of manufacture.
15. Expiry date of product.
16. Lot/batch number.
17. Storage condition

Pharmacovigilance of herbal medicinal products

The national government needs to strengthen capacity building in setting up and running such systems through training programmes, etc. While developing a national programme to monitor the safety of medicinal products, care should be taken to ensure that this will include:

1. Establishing a national pharmacovigilance center for monitoring the safety of medicinal products including herbal medicinal products.
2. Training staff that will be included in the reporting system.
3. Setting up necessary equipment.
4. Developing the reporting forms.
5. Setting up a multidisciplinary advisory committee to review and analyze the collected data.

Adverse drug reaction report

1. Pharmacovigilance units or national pharmacovigilance centers are necessary to collect and assess information on adverse drug reaction (ADR) relating to medicinal products including herbal medicines.
2. Where such units/centers exist, they should include herbal medicines in the current scope of their activities.
3. Each ADR report should be evaluated and assessed on the causality with the suspected herbal medicines.
4. Health professionals should be encouraged to ask their patients about the use of herbal products and herbal medicines, including 'medicinal foods/health food/dietary supplement' and any other medicines, and to include information on concomitant use in their ADR.
5. Each herbal medicine should be clearly identified by its constituents, brand name (if applicable) and dosage. If such information is missing in the ADR, the pharmacovigilance unit/center should immediately try to gather complete information, e.g. by asking the reporting health professional.

Pharmacovigilance units or national pharmacovigilance centers are necessary to collect and assess information on adverse drug reaction (ADR) relating to medicinal

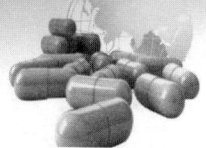

products including herbal medicines. Where such units/centers exist, they should include herbal medicines in the current scope of their activities.

1. Each ADR report should be evaluated and assessed on the causality with the suspected herbal medicines.
2. Health professionals should be encouraged to ask their patients about the use of herbal products and herbal medicines, including 'medicinal foods/health food/dietary supplement' and any other medicines, and to include information on concomitant use in their ADR.
3. Each herbal medicine should be clearly identified by its constituents, brand name (if applicable) and dosage. If such information is missing in the ADR, the pharmacovigilance unit/center should immediately try to gather complete information, e.g. by asking the reporting health professional.
4. To avoid the missing vital information, national drug regulation on herbal medicines and herbal medicines should include all the necessary information on registered herbal medicinal products and an ADR reporting form.

In analysing ADR reports the following aspects should be considered:

1. A literature search on the herbal product, its constituents and any co-medication should be performed.
2. The time—ADR relationship must be assessed:
   a. When did the ADR occur?
   b. Did the symptom occur when the herbal medication was started?
   c. Has any co-medication been used before the use of the herbal medicines without side-effect?
   d. Did the ADR occur when the co-medication was added to the herbal treatment?
   e. Did the ADR stop when the herbal medicines were withdrawn?
   f. Was the ADR reversible?
   g. Did the ADR reappear after re-exposure?
3. The dosage used should be compared with the traditional dosage described in the literature:
   a. Did the patient use a higher dose than recommended? Would it be intoxication rather than an ADR?
   b. Is the dosage so low compared to the traditional dose that a link is not plausible?
   c. Were there any signs of allergic reactions such as: rashes, asthma, eosinophilia, angioedema?
4. How common is the symptom with other diseases?
   a. What is the prevalence of diseases with the same symptoms, e.g. hepatitis?
   b. Can other causes be eliminated, such as viral markers or ethanol misuse in hepatitis?
   c. Search databases for similar case reports for association with the same or similar herbal medicines or combination products. In the case of suspicious

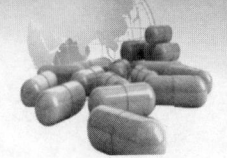

files, go to original reports, because the database file may not be complete and additional information may be found in the original report;

5. If no association was found in literature, or if an association is not plausible because of the low dose, there could be a problem related to the product's quality. Check for possible adulteration, substitution or contamination, e.g. by mycotoxins, heavy metals, etc.

The assessment should be done in cooperation with an expert panel comprising experts in pharmacognosy, toxicology and other health professionals including providers of herbal medicines. A clear conclusion on the causality should be made using the terms proposed by WHO Guidelines Related to Safety Drug Monitoring.

Reporting system on adverse events relating to herbal medicinal products

The following actions should be taken into account when setting up a reporting system, or including providers of herbal medicinal products in a pre-existing reporting system:

1. Provide education and awareness for the public/consumers and professionals including doctors, pharmacists, herbal medicine practitioners, etc.
2. Establish a proper regulatory system for herbal medicines.
3. Activate medicine information centers in health authorities for the establishment of special sections and systems for ADR of herbal medicines and any other possible medicine-related problem.
4. Use existing tools (for conventional drugs) to collect and analyse data supported by a computerized system.
5. Emphasize the scientific use of herbal medicines.
6. Solve existing problems in the reporting systems by using advanced database programmes.
7. Ask for WHO assistance in establishing an ADR reporting system.
8. Encourage manufacturers, the public/consumers and professionals including doctors, pharmacists, practitioners of herbal medicine, etc. who produce, prescribe or use herbal medicines, to report ADR to relevant authorities.

Control of advertisements of herbal medicinal products

The national authorities responsible for the regulation of herbal medicinal products and practices should approve every advertisement before it reaches the public. The regulatory authority should issue advertisement permits after satisfactory evaluation of the contents of each advertisement to ensure that the public gets the correct information about the product, devoid of ambiguous or fraudulent claims. The print and electronic media should be notified to ensure that every advertiser of herbal medicinal products obtains the permit from the national authority before such an advertisement is published.

It is necessary that information on the advertisement of herbal medicinal products is shared among countries and overall cooperation with different, relevant national authorities is encouraged.

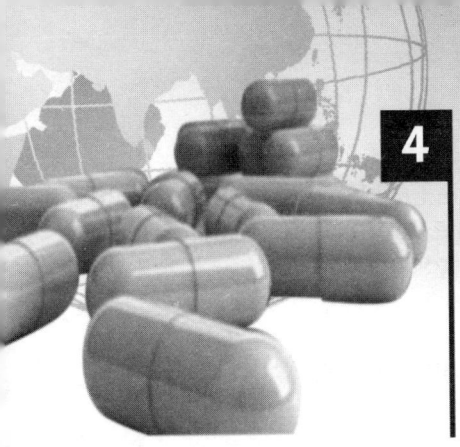

International Conference on Harmonization

4

INTRODUCTION

The "International conference on harmonization (ICH) of technical requirements for the Registration of Pharmaceuticals for human use. To assure safety, quality and efficacy of medicines, the members of ICH include members from drug regulatory authorities and research based industries of the European Union, the US and Japan will discuss on the technical procedures and documents required. It is unique project that brings together the regulatory authorities and pharmaceutical industry of Europe, Japan and the US to discuss scientific and technical aspects of drug registration. It was formed to achieve greater harmonization in the interpretation and application of technical guidelines and requirements for pharmaceutical product registration in the EU, Japan and the USA.

In simple words *"ICH has been framed to have a common scientific and technical requirements for registration of pharmaceuticals in the EU, Japan and the USA to make the job easy for regulatory agencies and pharma companies"*.

Origin of ICH

Harmonization of regulatory requirements was pioneered by the European Community (EC), in the 1980s, as the EC (now the European Union) moved towards the development of a single market for pharmaceuticals. The success achieved in Europe demonstrated that harmonization was feasible. At the same time there were bilateral discussions between Europe, Japan and the US on possibilities for harmonization. It was, however, at the WHO Conference of Drug Regulatory Authorities (ICDRA), in Paris, in 1989, that specific plans for action began to materialize. Soon afterwards, the authorities approached IFPMA to discuss a joint regulatory-industry initiative on international harmonization, and ICH was conceived.

The birth of ICH took place at a meeting in April 1990, hosted by EFPIA in Russels. Representatives of the regulatory agencies and industry associations of Europe, Japan and the US met, primarily, to plan an International Conference but the meeting also discussed the wider implications and terms of reference of ICH. At the first ICH Steering Committee (SC) meeting of ICH the Terms of Reference

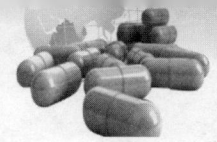

were agreed and it was decided that the Topics selected for harmonization would be divided into safety, quality and efficacy to reflect the three criteria which are the basis for approving and authorising new medicinal products.

Benefits of ICH

Harmonization is beneficial to both regulatory authorities and the pharmaceutical industry, ultimately having beneficial impact for the protection of public health. The benefits of harmonization are listed below.

1. Promote international harmonization of technical requirements to develop safe, effective, and high quality medicines.
2. Reduce the registration cost.
3. Promote public health.
4. Prevent the duplication of clinical trials in humans.
5. Minimize the animal use without compromising in the safety, quality of the product.
6. Promote international harmonization by bringing together representatives from the three ICH regions (the EU, Japan and the USA) to discuss and establish common guidelines.
7. Make information available on ICH, ICH activities and ICH guidelines to any country.

ICH Secretariat

ICH does not have "offices" as such, but **ICH secretariat is based in Geneva**, Switzerland. The biannual meetings and conferences of the ICH Steering Committee rotate between the EU, Japan, and the USA.

Members of ICH

ICH is comprised of representatives from six parties that represent the regulatory bodies and research based industry in the European Union, Japan and the USA.

1. In Japan, the members are the Ministry of Health, Labour and Welfare (MHLW), and the Japan Pharmaceutical Manufacturers Association (JPMA). In Europe, the members are the European Union (EU), and the European Federation of Pharmaceutical Industries and Associations (EFPIA).
2. In the USA, the members are the Food and Drug Administration (FDA), and the Pharmaceutical Research and Manufacturers of America (PhRMA).
3. Additional members include observers from the World Health Organization (WHO), European Free Trade Association (EFTA), Canada.

Voting Members in ICH

Members from Japan:
- Ministry of Health, Labour and Welfare (MHLW)
- Japan Pharmaceutical Manufacturers Association (JPMA).

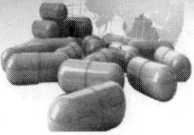

Members from Europe:
• European Union (EU)
• European Federation of Pharmaceutical Industries and Associations (EFPIA).

Members from the USA:
• Food and Drug Administration (FDA)
• Pharmaceutical Research and Manufacturers

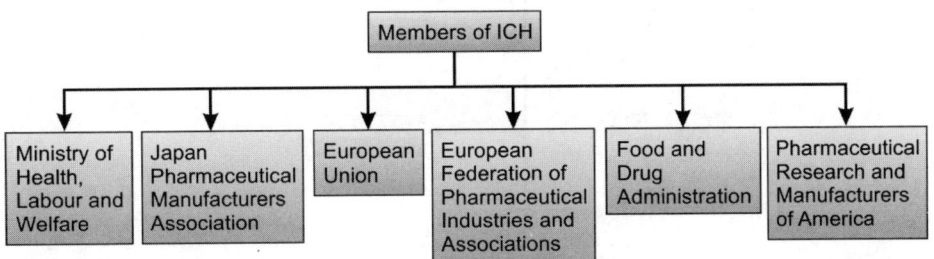

Figure 4.1 shows non-voting member of ICH

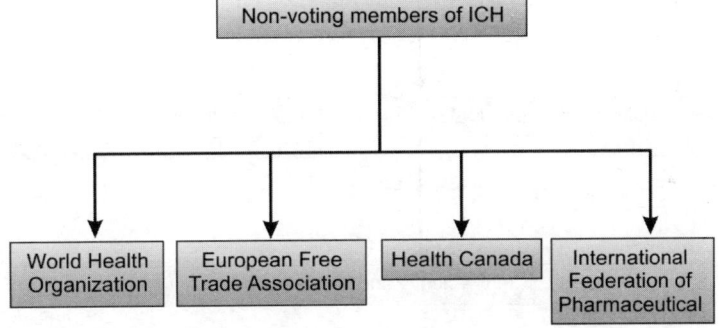

Fig. 4.1: Figure showing non-voting members of ICH

WHO: World Health Organization
EFTA: European Free Trade Association
IFPMA: International Federation of Pharmaceutical Manufacturers and Associations

Responsibilities of Non-voting Members of ICH

1. Provides support to the ICH Steering Committee.
2. Documents the meetings of the Steering Committee.
3. Promotes coordination between working groups.
4. Provides information on the ICH guidelines and ICH process.
5. Provides administrative support for MedDRA management board.
6. Provides administrative support for global cooperation group

Organization of ICH (Fig. 4.2)

The organizational structure of ICH consists of the following components:

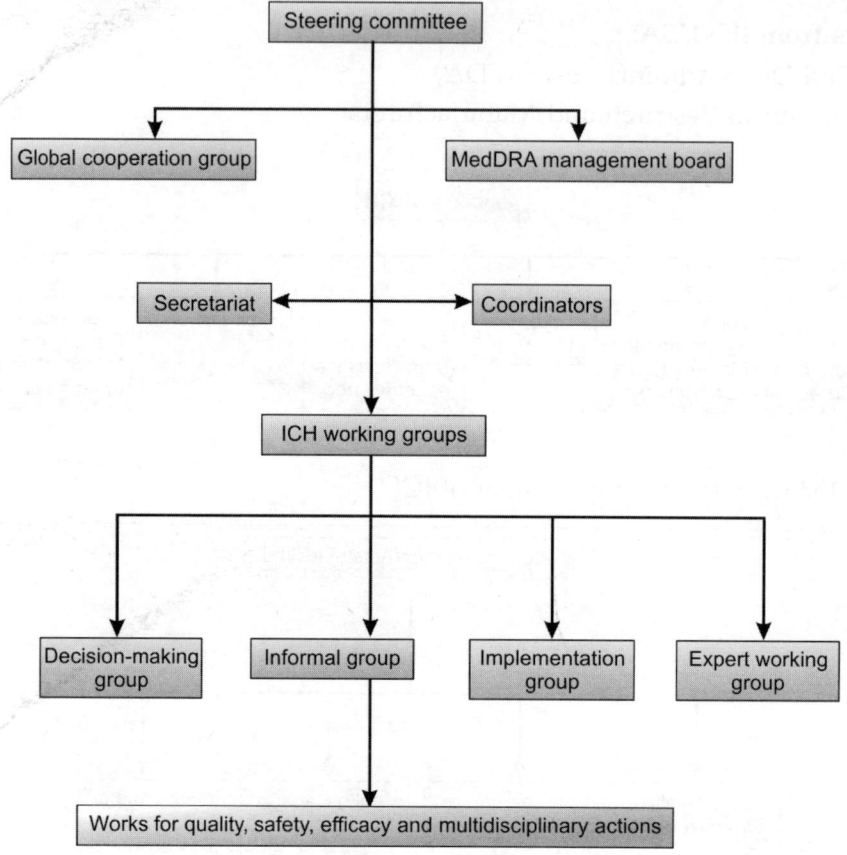

Fig. 4.2: Organization of ICH

Responsibilities of ICH steering committee

The ICH Steering Committee (SC) is the main organization which is involved in the following works:

   i. Governs ICH
  ii. Determines the policies and procedures for ICH.
 iii. Selects topics for harmonization
  iv. Monitors the progress of harmonization initiatives

Process of Harmonization

ICH harmonization activities fall into 4 categories: Formal ICH procedure, Q&A procedure, revision procedure and maintenance procedure, depending on the activity to be undertaken in Fig. 4.3.

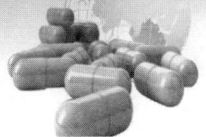

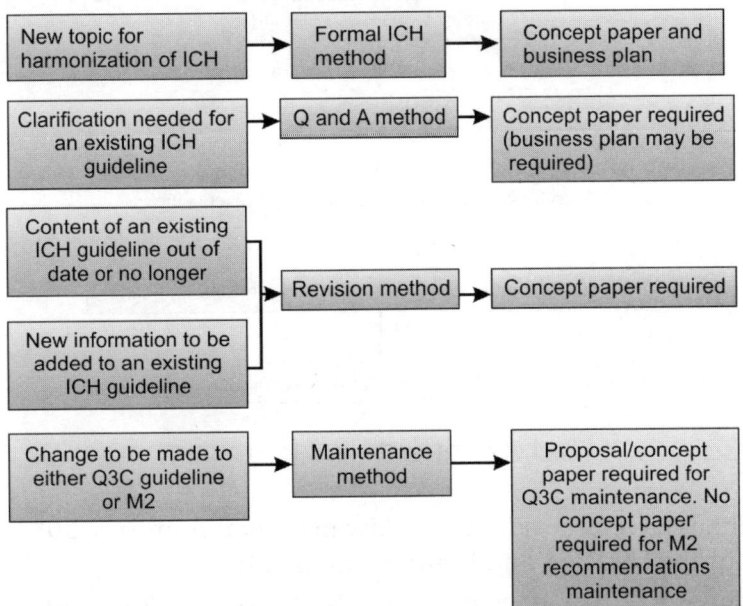

Fig. 4.3: Process of harmonization

Steps Involved in the ICH Procedure

Step 1: Drafts are prepared and circulated through many revisions until a "final harmonized draft" is completed under the leadership of the Rapporteur.

Step 2: This draft is signed by the expert working group (EWG) as the agreed-upon draft and forwarded to the Steering Committee for signing which signifies acceptance for consultation by each of the six co-sponsors.

Step 3: The three regulatory sponsors initiate their normal consultation process to receive comments. This comment period normally takes six months. The draft document to be generated as a result of the Step 3 phase is called Step 4 experts document. If both regulatory and industry parties of the EWG are satisfied that the consensus achieved at Step 2 is not substantially altered as a result of the consultation, or consensus is reached on any alterations, the Step 4 experts document is signed by the EWG regulatory experts. The Step 4 document with regulatory EWG signatures is submitted to the Steering Committee to request adoption as Step 4 of the ICH process.

Step 4: It is reached when the Steering Committee agrees that there is sufficient scientific consensus on the technical issues. This endorsement is based on the signatures from the three regulatory parties to ICH affirming that the guideline is recommended for adoption by the regulatory bodies of the three regions.

Step 5: The process is complete when the guidelines are incorporated into national or regional internal procedures in Fig. 4.4.

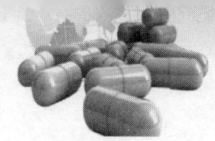

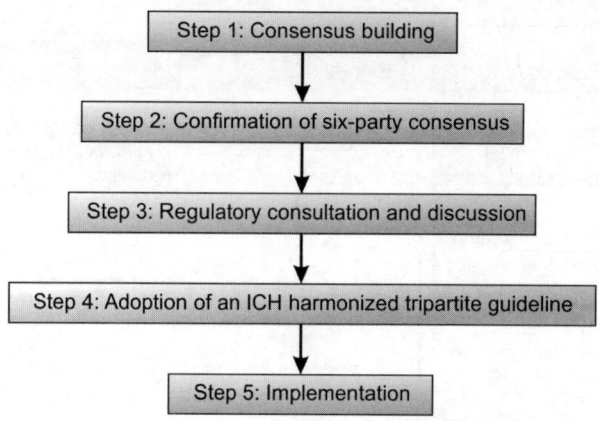

Fig. 4.4: Steps involve in ICH procedure

ICH guidelines have been adopted as law in several countries, but are only used as guidance for the US Food and Drug Administration.

The guidelines of ICH may be broadly categorized into four types:

1. Quality guidelines
2. Safety guidelines
3. Efficacy guidelines
4. Multidisciplinary guidelines

Quality guidelines: Harmonization achievements in the quality area include pivotal milestones such as the conduct of stability studies, defining relevant thresholds for impurities testing and a more flexible approach to pharmaceutical quality based on good manufacturing practice (GMP) risk management.

Safety guidelines: ICH has produced a comprehensive set of safety guidelines to uncover potential risks like carcinogenicity, genotoxicity and reprotoxicity. A recent breakthrough has been a non-clinical testing strategy for assessing the QT interval prolongation liability: The single most important cause of drug withdrawals in recent years.

Efficacy guidelines: The work carried out by ICH under the efficacy heading is concerned with the design, conduct, safety and reporting of clinical trials. It also covers novel types of medicines derived from biotechnological processes and the use of pharmacogenetics/genomics techniques to produce better targeted medicines.

Multidisciplinary guidelines: Those are the cross-cutting topics which do not fit uniquely into one of the quality, safety and efficacy categories. It includes the ICH medical terminology (MedDRA), the Common Technical Document (CTD) and the development of Electronic Standards for the Transfer of Regulatory Information (ESTRI).

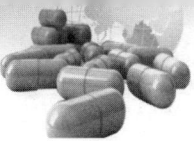

Q: Quality guidelines

Q1a–Q1f	*Stability studies*
Q1a	Stability testing of new drug substances and products
Q1b	Photostability testing of new drug substances and products
Q1c	Stability testing of new dosage forms
Q1d	Bracketing and matrixing designs for stability testing of new drug substances and products
Q1e	Evaluation of stability data
Q1f	Stability data packages for registration in climatic zone iii and iv
Q2a	Validation of analytical procedures
Q2b	Methodology
Q3a-Q3d	Impurities
Q3a	Impurity testing in new drug substance
Q3b	Impurities in dosage form
Q3c	Impurities in residual solvent
Q3d	Guidelines for metal impurities
Q4	Pharmacopoeial harmonization
Q5a-Q5d	Quality of biotechnology products
Q5a	Viral safety evaluation
Q5b	Genetic stability
Q5c	Stability of biotechnology products
Q5d	Stability of cell substances
Q6	Specifications for new drug substances and products
Q7	Good manufacturing practice
Q8	Pharmaceutical development
Q9	Quality risk management
Q10	Pharmaceutical quality system

Safety guidelines

E1	Clinical safety for drugs intended for long-term treatment of non-life-threatening conditions
E2a	Clinical safety data management
E2b(R5)	Implementation working group questions and answers
E2b(R2)	Maintenance of ICH guidline on clinical safety
E2c(R1)	Clinical safety and periodic safety for marketed drugs
E2d	Post-approval safety data management

Contd.

Contd.

E2e	Pharmacovigilance planning
E2f	Development safety update report
E3	Structure and content of clinical study reports
E4	Dose-response information to support drug registration
E5	Implementation working group questions and answers
E5(R1)	Ethnic factors in the acceptability of foreign clinical data
E6 (R1)	Guideline for good clinical practice
E7	Studies in support of special populations: questions and answers
E8	Statistical principles for clinical trials
E9	Statistical principles for clinical trials
E10	Choice of control group and related issues in clinical trials
E11	Clinical investigation of medicinal products in the pediatric population
E12	Clinical evaluation of new anti-hypertensive drugs
E14	Clinical evaluation for non-antiarrhythmic potential
E15	Biomarkers related to drug for biotechnology product development
E16	Biomarkers related to drug for biotechnology product development

Multidisciplinary guidelines

M2(R2)	Electronic transmission of individual case safety reports message specification
M3(R3)	Guidance on non-clinical safety studies for the conduct of human clinical trials and marketing authorization for pharmaceuticals
M4	Organization of the common technical document for the registration of pharmaceutical for human use
M4e(R1)	The common technical document for the registration of pharmaceuticals for human use: Efficacy
M4q(R1)	The common technical document for the registration of pharmaceuticals for human use: Quality
M4s(R2)	The common technical document for the registration of pharmaceuticals for human use: Safety
M5	Data elements and standards for drug dictionaries

The Impact of ICH (Efficacy) on Industry

1. Repeat clinical trials were a fact of life in drug development if a company wished to market a drug in more than one region. This costly and time consuming activity, frequently involving the repeat of long, resource intensive Phase III clinical trials, is obviated in most cases by the introduction of ethnic factors in the acceptability of foreign clinical data" (E5) guideline.

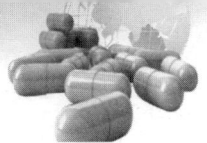

2. When the trials are run in accordance with the principles of GCP laid down in the ICH guideline "Good Clinical Practice: Consolidated Guideline" (E6), foreign clinical trial data may be submitted in support of a submission in any ICH region.

3. Less than a year after the guideline was finalized Pfizer was able to apply it to great effect to gain approval of Viagra® in Japan by use of a bridging study (a key part of the E5 guideline), rather than a repeated clinical trial(s) as would have been required previously.

4. The guideline "General Considerations for Clinical Trials" (E8), provides a set of internationally accepted principles to be applied to trial design, which aids the acceptance of data throughout the three regions.

5. The guideline E2A (Clinical Safety Data Management: Definitions and standards for expedited reporting) and E3 (Structure and Content of Clinical Study Reports). E2A led to a harmonization of expedited reporting in the three regions, defining when clinical study reports are required and the amount of detail they should contain. It also ensures that reporting times are measured in calendar days rather than working days.

6. E3 (Clinical Study Reports), like E6 (GCP), early ICH process, establishing a common format for clinical study reports. This common presentation has made preparing multiple regulatory submissions a far simpler process as a single core document (with appendices) may be used in all three ICH regions.

7. One of the most important outcomes of the harmonization work in the efficacy area, as well as the recognized reduction in time and resources used in a development program, is that the unified operating practices enhanced patient safety in the clinical trials process.

The Impact of ICH (Quality) on Industry

1. The ICH guidelines in the Quality area have provided recommendations in two of the key areas that define bulk drug and drug product quality—stability data and impurities—and led to a significant reduction in duplicate testing.

2. Prior to these guidelines there was no harmonized approach to the data requirements in these areas. With stability for example, it was typical to run studies at "room temperature" as defined by the company concerned, and appropriate to the locality.

3. There was also no humidity control. This resulted in registrations in different regions requiring new stability data if the climatic zone was different to that where the original study had been conducted.

4. ICH harmonization provided standard sets of conditions taking account of the climatic zones in each of the three regions.

5. This means that the information on stability generated in any one of the three regions is mutually acceptable in the other two areas, provided it meets the requirements of the guideline. This removed the duplicate testing.

6. The impurities guidelines (Impurities in New Drug Substances (Q3A), Impurities in New Drug Products (Q3B), and Impurities: Guideline for Residual Solvents (Q3C)) also served, as with the stability guidelines, to provide scientific agreement on the recording and reporting of impurity levels.

7. Guidelines were also provided on how changes in impurity profile over the course of a development program should be managed. The result of this is that it should be possible to determine a single specification for any drug substance or product that is acceptable across the three ICH regions. This makes the supply chain far simpler, and minimizes supply error.

8. ICH has also produced a parallel set of guidelines covering the specific issues associated with biotechnological products. Standardization through the guidelines has been a very positive step for the biotechnology industry, and has certainly had a significant favorable impact on both development times and resource utilization.

9. Duplication of research was reduced related to the stability testing, impurity profiles.

The Impact of ICH (Safety) on Industry

1. The guidelines in this area have very much represented industry's current best practice.

2. By a careful examination of standard practice and the types of data that could be accessed from studies the EWGs in this area were able to determine what testing was necessary to examine any one type of toxicity, and thus to generate a standard battery of tests.

3. This resulted in the guidelines comprehensively covering carcinogenicity testing, genotoxicity testing, reprotoxicity testing, chronic toxicity testing.

4. There is also a guideline concerning biotechnology derived pharmaceuticals, and guideline for the timing of non-clinical safety studies for the conduct of human clinical trials for pharmaceuticals (M3). This defined the safety data that must be available before human volunteers or patients may be treated with the new drug.

5. There is a standard set of tests recommended for most types of toxicity studies; timing, exact requirements (including dose) and need for toxicity studies for different indications or treatment durations have been defined.

6. For carcinogenicity studies only one long-term study (usually carried out in a rodent species) plus one short- or mid-term study is needed. The safety guidelines made long-term studies easy.

7. Currently, with the results available at the end of 2000; the special case of biotechnological products has also been considered. All of these resulted in a reduction in duplicate testing.

8. As safety testing is an area of considerable research effort, both in academia and industry, an important result of, for example, the reduction in the number of long term studies that is required should be that (as well as reducing the

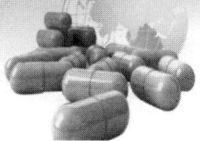

use of animals) it will allow more resource to be diverted to other approaches to uncover potential risks like genotoxicity and carcinogenicity relevant to humans.

9. The continual development of the models used to study toxicity is key to the industry becoming better able to evaluate the safety of new drugs, and delivering safe therapies to patients.

10. It is on the basis of such research developments that ICH tries to keep guidelines updated and under review.

Conclusion

ICH, through its activities in the harmonization of regulatory requirements across the EU, Japan and the US, is enabling industry to reduce development times by removing the duplication of studies that was previously required to gain market approval for a new drug in each of the three regions. Industry has three reasons to support ICH and its continued efforts to further harmonize the technical requirements for the registration of innovative drugs which are reduced development times and resources, including an end to duplicate clinical trials due to ethnicity differences, easier simultaneous launch of a new drug in many countries (including across the three ICH regions), ICH guidelines as a recognized standard, will facilitate intra-company globalization. Harmonization through ICH brings important, life-saving treatments to patients faster.

COMMON TECHNICAL DOCUMENT

Introduction

Common technical document (CTD) is a format that was created by the ICH (International Conference on Harmonization) in an attempt to harmonize the format of drug approval's applications in all 3 ICH regions, i.e. the USA, Europe and Japan. The CTD was agreed upon in November 2000, in San Diego, California, the USA.

CTD is a common format/template to provide the information to the Drug Regulatory authorities in the 3 ICH regions. It is not a "single" dossier, with a "single" content since legal requirements and applicant preferences differ in the 3 different ICH regions.

The CTD as defined by the ICH M4 expert working group (EWG) does not cover the full submission that is to be made in a region. It describes only modules 2 to 5, which are common across all regions. The CTD does not describe the content of module 1, the regional administrative information and prescribing information, nor does it describe documents that can be submitted as amendments or variations to the initial application.

The CTD is a set of specifications for the submission of regulatory data in the application for obtaining market approval for pharmaceuticals. The format of the CTD is not to be confused with its content or submission type; rather, it is the means by which information in a submission is organized.

Specification for the organization of content of CTD

For modules 2–5 (excluding the regional section within module 3, i.e. 3.2 R), the ICH specifies the organization and content for CTD. For regional sections (Module 1 and the regional section within Module 3), the specific regulatory authority (i.e. FDA, Singapore, Health Canada and India) specifies the organization and content for CTD, therefore regional section content may vary between different ICH regions.

Objective of ICH behind CTD

1. To present a well-structured common format for the preparation of approval's applications which will be submitted to regulatory authorities.
2. To significantly reduce the time and resources needed to compile applications for registration of human pharmaceuticals and ease the preparation of electronic submissions.
3. To facilitate the regulatory reviews and communication with the applicant by using a standard document of common elements.
4. To prevent unnecessary duplication of work.

In addition, exchange of regulatory information between regulatory authorities will be simplified, i.e. faster availability of new medicines.

Table 4.1 shows the implementation dates of CTD.

Table 4.1: Implementation Dates of CTD	
Optional, July 2001	EU, FDA, MHLW (as well as Canada and Switzerland)
Mandatory, July 2003	EU, MHLW (as well as Canada* and Switzerland*) Non-ICH countries
Highly recommended, July 2003	FDA

* These are non-ICH countries but have accepted to adopt CTD format for application.

Benefits of the CTD

1. Complete, well-organized submissions
2. More predictable format
3. More consistent reviews
4. Easier analysis across applications
5. Easier exchange of information
6. Facilitates electronic submissions

Organization of the Common Technical Document

The common technical document is organized into five modules (Table 4.2).

Objectives of CTD Guideline

This guideline is intended to provide recommendations on how to use stability data generated in accordance with the principles detailed in the ICH guideline Q1A(R) stability testing of new drug substances and products (here after referred

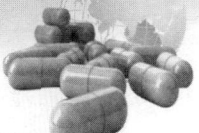

Table 4.2: Modules of common technical document	
Module 1	A regional specific module containing administrative information, and is unique to each regulatory authority
Module 2	Contains overviews, written summaries and tabulated summaries of the data contained in modules 3, 4 and 5
Module 3	Contains quality data relating to the drug substance and drug product
Module 4	Contains nonclinical data
Module 5	Contains clinical data

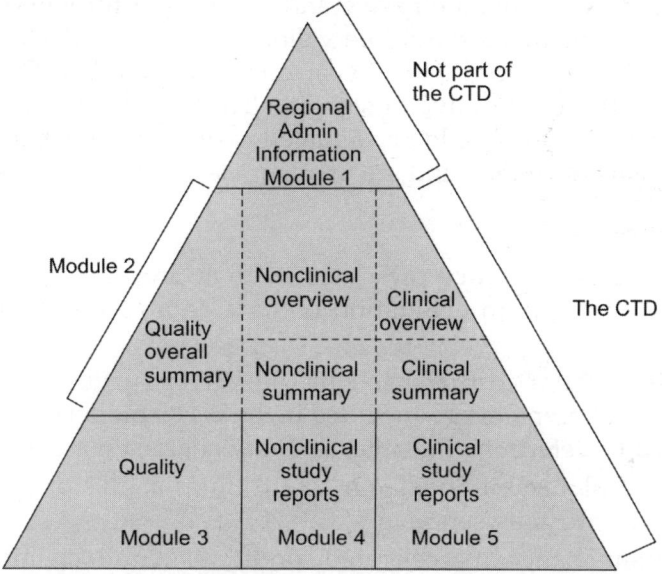

Fig. 4.5: Diagrammatic presentation of CTD modules

as the parent guideline) to propose a retest period/shelf life in a registration application in Fig. 4.5.

This guideline describes when and how extrapolation can be considered when proposing a retest period for a drug substance or a shelf life for a drug product that extends beyond the period covered by available data from the stability study under the long-term storage condition (hereafter referred to as long-term data).

Background

The guidance on the evaluation and statistical analysis of stability data provided in the parent guideline is brief in nature and limited in scope. The parent guideline states that regression analysis is an appropriate approach to analyze quantitative stability data for retest period or shelf life estimation and recommends that a statistical test for batch poolability be performed using a level of significance of 0.25. However, the parent guideline includes few details and does not cover situations where multiple factors are involved in a full- or reduced-design study.

General Principles

The design and execution of formal stability studies should follow the principles outlined in the parent guideline. A systematic approach should be adopted to the presentation and evaluation of stability information, which should include, as necessary, physical, chemical, biological and microbiological test characteristics. All product characteristics likely to be affected by storage, e.g. assay value or potency, content of products of decomposition, physicochemical properties (hardness, disintegration, particulate matter, etc.), should be determined; for solid or semi-solid oral dosage forms, dissolution tests should be carried out. Test methods to demonstrate the efficacy of additives, such as antimicrobial agents, should be used to determine whether such additives remain effective and unchanged throughout the projected shelf-life. Analytical methods should be validated or verified, and the accuracy as well as the precision (standard deviations) should be recorded. The assay methods chosen should be those indicative of stability. The tests for related compounds or products of decomposition should be validated to demonstrate that they are specific to the product being examined and are of adequate sensitivity.

Data Presentation

Data for all attributes should be presented in an appropriate format (e.g. tabular, graphical, narrative) and an evaluation of such data should be included in the application.

1. A checklist similar to that used in the WHO survey on the stability of pharmaceutical preparations included in the WHO model list of essential drugs can be used to determine the other stability characteristics of the product.
2. Tabulate and plot stability data on all attributes at all storage conditions and evaluate each attribute separately.
3. No significant change at accelerated conditions within six months.
4. Long-term data show little or no variability and little or no change over time.

Stability Protocol and Report

1. Batches tested
2. General information
3. Container/closure system
4. Literature and supporting data
5. Stability-indicating analytical methods
6. Testing plan
7. Test parameters
8. Test results
9. Other requirements (post-approval commitments)
10. Conclusion

Result sheets must bear date and responsible person signature/QA approval and the batches should be representative of the manufacturing process and should be manufactured from different batches of key intermediates (Table 4.3).

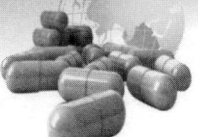

Table 4.3: Illustrative data of capsule/tablet stability batches			
Batch number			
Date of manufacture			
Site of manufacture			
Batch size (kg)	20	100	100
Batch size (number of units)			
Primary packing materials			
Date of initial analysis			
Batch number of the API			

Extrapolation

1. Extrapolation is the practice of using a known data set to infer information about future data.
2. Extrapolation to extend the retest period or shelf life beyond the period covered by long-term data can be proposed in the application, particularly if no significant change is observed at the accelerated condition.

Data evaluation for retest period or shelf life estimation for drug substances or products intended for room temperature storage.

No significant change at accelerated condition

Where no significant change occurs at the accelerated condition, the retest period or shelf life would depend on the nature of the long-term and accelerated data (Fig. 4.6).

Significant change at accelerated condition

Where significant change occurs at the accelerated condition, the retest period or shelf life would depend on the outcome of stability testing at the intermediate condition, as well as at the long-term condition.

The following physical changes can be expected to occur at the accelerated condition and would not be considered significant change that calls for intermediate testing if there is no other significant change:

1. Softening of a suppository that is designed to melt at 37°C, if the melting point is clearly demonstrated.
2. Failure to meet acceptance criteria for dissolution for 12 units of a gelatin capsule or gel-coated tablet if the failure can be unequivocally attributed to cross-linking.

However, if phase separation of a semi-solid dosage form occurs at the accelerated condition, testing at the intermediate condition should be performed. Potential interaction effects should also be considered in establishing that there is no other significant change.

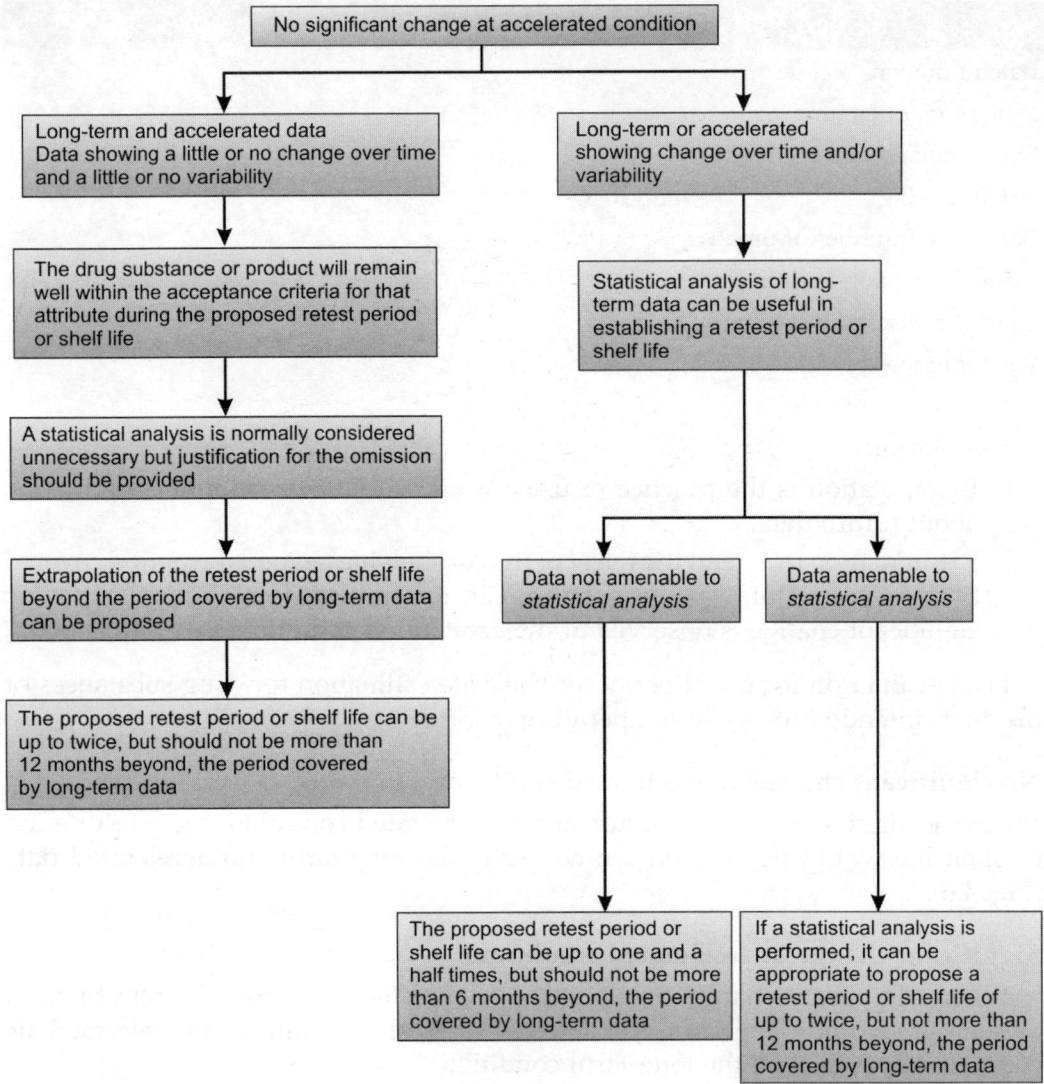

Fig. 4.6: Showing no significant change at accelerated study significant change at accelerated condition

Data evaluation for product intended for storage below room temperature

1. Drug substances or products intended for storage in a refrigerator
2. Drug substances or products intended for storage in a freezer
3. Drug substances or products intended for storage below –20°C

General Statistical Approaches

Where applicable, an appropriate statistical method should be employed to analyze the long-term primary stability data in an original application.

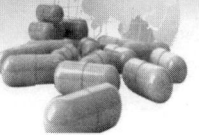

1. The purpose of this analysis is to establish, with a high degree of confidence, a retest period or shelf life during which a quantitative attribute will remain within acceptance criteria for all future batches manufactured, packaged, and stored under similar circumstances.

2. The same statistical method should also be used to analyze data from commitment batches to verify or extend the originally approved retest period or shelf life.

3. **Regression analysis** is considered an appropriate approach to evaluating the stability data for a quantitative attribute and establishing a retest period or shelf life.

4. The relationship between **an attribute and time** can be **represented by a linear or non-linear function on an arithmetic or logarithmic scale.**

5. In some cases, a non-linear regression can better reflect the true relationship.

6. An appropriate approach to retest period or shelf life estimation is to analyze a quantitative attribute (e.g. assay, degradation products) by **determining the earliest time at which the 95 percent confidence limit for the mean intersects the proposed acceptance criterion.**

7. For an attribute known to decrease with time, the lower one-sided 95 percent confidence limit should be compared to the acceptance criterion.

8. For an attribute known to increase with time, the upper one-sided 95 percent confidence limit should be compared to the acceptance criterion.

9. For an attribute that can either increase or decrease, or whose direction of change is not known, two-sided 95 percent confidence limits should be calculated and compared to the upper and lower acceptance criteria (Fig. 4.7).

Stability data package for registration in Climatic Zones III and IV.

Objectives of the Guideline

This guideline describes outlines the stability data package for a new drug substance or drug product that is considered sufficient for a registration application in territories in Climatic Zones III and IV.

Background

A product's shelf life should be established according to climatic conditions in which the product is to be marketed. Storage conditions recommended by manufacturers on the basis of stability studies are meant to guarantee the maintenance of quality, safety and efficacy throughout the shelf-life of product. Temperature and humidity determine the storage conditions and so they greatly affect the stability of drug product. Climatic conditions in countries where the product is to be marketed should be carefully considered during drug development phase. So the world has been divided into four climatic zones based on prevalent annual climatic conditions.

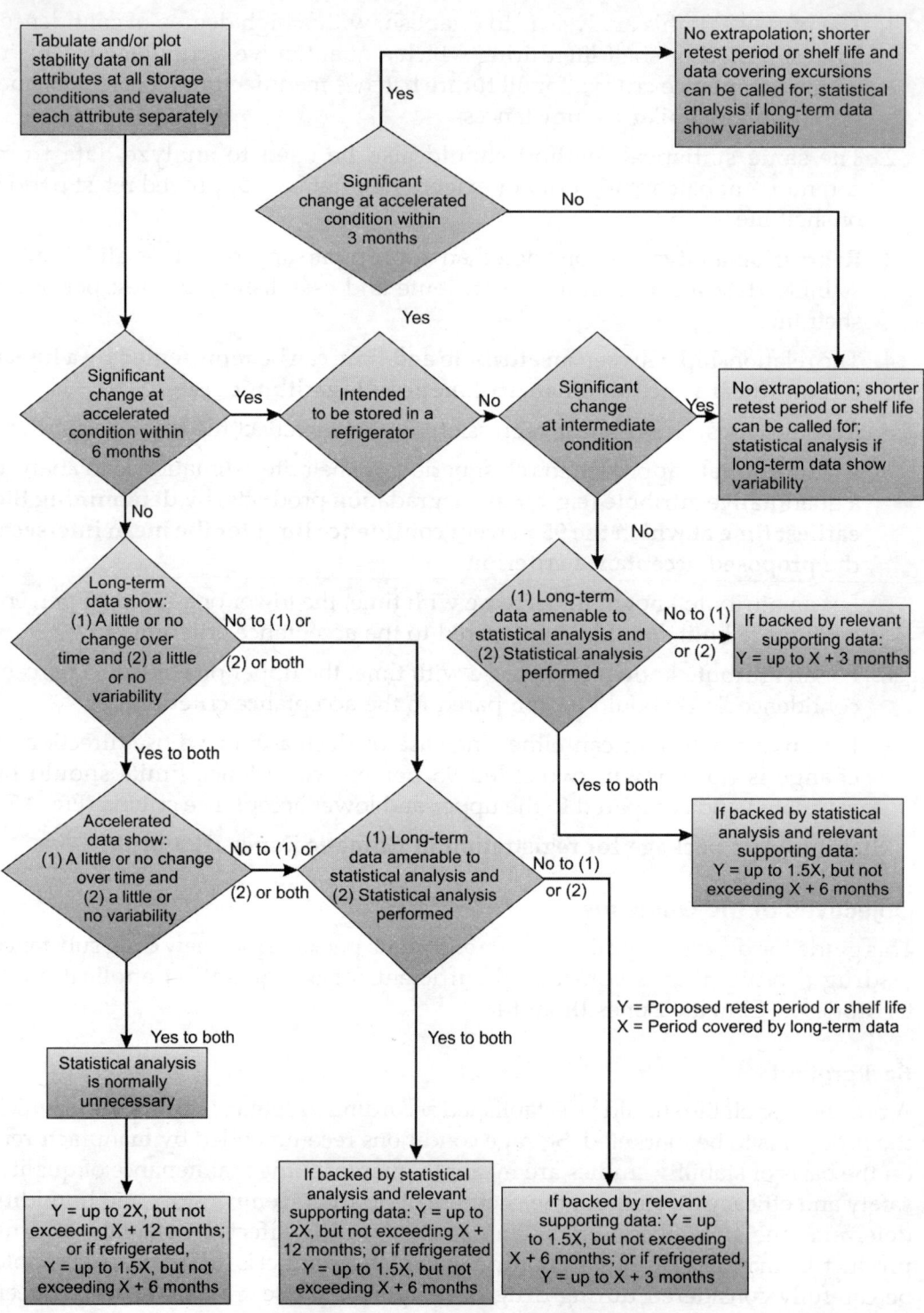

Fig. 4.7: General statistical approaches

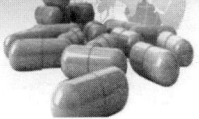

Definition and Storage/Test Conditions for Four Climatic Zones

Climatic zones	Definition	Storage/test conditios	Examples
I	Temperate climate	21°C ± 2°C and 45% RH ± 5% RH	Northern Europe, Canada
II	Mediterranean and subtropical climate	25°C ± 2°C and 60% RH ± 5% RH	Southern Europe, Japan, US
III	Hot dry climate	30°C ± 2°C and 35% RH ± 5% RH	Egypt, Sudan
IV	Hot and humid climate	30°C ± 2°C and 75% RH ± 5% RH	Central Africa, South Pacific

SCOPE OF THE GUIDELINE

This document is an annex to the parent guideline and recommends the long-term storage condition for stability testing of a new drug substance or drug product for a registration application in territories in Climatic Zones III and IV.

Guidelines

Continuity with the Parent Guideline

The following sections of the parent guideline can be considered common to any territory in the world and are not reproduced here: Stress testing, selection of batches, container closure system, specification, testing frequency, storage conditions for drug substance or product in a refrigerator, storage conditions for drug substance or product in a freezer, stability commitment, evaluation, statements/labeling.

Storage Conditions

General Case

For the general case (as described in the parent guideline), the recommended long-term and accelerated storage conditions for Climatic Zones III and IV are shown in Table 4.4.

Table 4.4: Storage condition for general case		
Type of study	**Storage condition**	**Minimum time period covered by data at submission**
Long-term	30°C ± 2°C/65% RH ± 5% RH	12 months
Accelerated	40°C ± 2°C/75% RH ± 5% RH	6 months

No intermediate storage condition for stability studies is recommended for Climatic Zones III and IV. Thus, the intermediate storage condition is not relevant when the principles of retest period or shelf life extrapolation described in Q1E are applied.

Aqueous-based drug products packaged in semi-permeable containers

For aqueous-based drug products packaged in semi-permeable containers (as described in the parent guideline), the recommended long-term and accelerated storage conditions for Climatic Zones III and IV are shown in Table 4.5.

Table 4.5: Aqueous-based drug products packaged in semi-permeable containers		
Type of study	Storage condition	Minimum time period covered by data at submission
Long-term	30 °C ± 2 °C/35% RH ± 5% RH	12 months
Accelerated	40 °C ± 2 °C/ Not more than 25% RH ± 5% RH	6 months

As described in the parent guideline, an appropriate approach for deriving the water loss rate at the reference relative humidity is to multiply the water loss rate measured at an alternative relative humidity at the same temperature by a water loss rate ratio (Table 4.6).

The ratio of water loss rates at a given temperature is calculated by the general formula (100 − reference % RH)/(100 − alternative % RH).

Table 4.6: Alternate relative humidity and reference relative humidity for aqueous based products		
Alternative relative humidity	Reference relative humidity	Ratio of water loss rates at a given temperature
65% RH	35% RH	1.9
75% RH	25% RH	3.0

Valid water loss rate ratios at relative humidity conditions other than those shown in the table above can be used. A linear water loss rate at the alternative relative humidity over the storage period should be demonstrated.

Tests at elevated temperature and/or extremes of humidity

Special transportation and climatic conditions outside the storage conditions recommended in this guideline should be supported by additional data. For example, these data can be obtained from studies on one batch of drug product conducted for up to 3 months at 50 °C/ambient humidity to cover extremely hot and dry conditions and at 25 °C/80% RH to cover extremely high humidity conditions.

Stability testing at a high humidity condition, e.g. 25°C/80% RH is recommended for solid dosage forms in water-vapor permeable packaging, e.g. tablets in PVC/ aluminum blisters, intended to be marketed in territories with extremely high humidity conditions in Zone IV. However, for solid dosage forms in primary

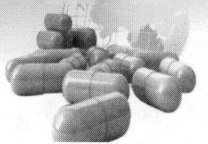

containers designed to provide a barrier to water vapor, e.g. aluminum/aluminum blisters, stability testing at a storage condition of extremely high humidity is not considered necessary.

Additional Considerations

If it cannot be demonstrated that the drug substance or drug product will remain within its acceptance criteria when stored at 30 °C ± 2 °C/65 % RH ± 5 % RH for the duration of the proposed retest period or shelf life, the following options should be considered: (1) a reduced retest period or shelf life, (2) a more protective container closure system, or (3) additional cautionary statements in the labeling.

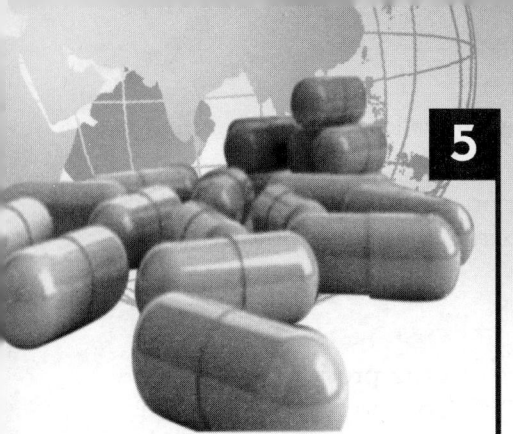

Orphan Drugs

In the USA, orphan drugs are defined as "those intended for the safe and effective treatment, diagnosis or prevention of rare diseases/disorders that affect very few among 200,000 people in the US. Hence, it is not expected to recover the costs of developing and marketing a treatment drug".

In the EU, orphan drugs are defined as "those that are intended for diagnosis, prevention or treatment of diseases that affect fewer than 5 in 10,000 people across the EU".

In simple words "Orphan drugs are those, which are intended for the treatment of rare diseases".

Definition of Orphan Drugs in Different Countries

United States: In the US, any drug developed under the Orphan Drug Act of January 1983 (ODA) is an orphan drug. The ODA is a federal law concerning rare diseases (orphan diseases) that affect fewer than 200,000 people in the United States or are of low prevalence (less than 5 per 10,000 in the community).

Europe: A disease or disorder that affects fewer than 5 in 10,000 citizens (Orphan Drug Regulation 141/2000). According to European Organization for Rare Diseases (EURORDIS), the number of rare diseases numbers from about 6,000 to 8,000, most of which have identified genetic conditions, with medical literature describing approximately five new rare conditions every week. Twenty-five to Thirty million people are reported to be affected by these diseases in Europe.

Japan: Any disease with fewer than 50,000 prevalent cases (0.4%) is Japan's definition of rare. The drug treats a disease or condition for which there are no other treatments available in Japan or the proposed drug is clinically superior to drugs already available on the Japanese market. The applicant should have a clear product development plan and scientific rationale to support the necessity of the drug in Japan. Once clinical trials are completed, a New Drug Application (NDA) can be submitted. It is important to keep in mind that while Japan has orphan drug legislation, this legislation has room for interpretation.

Few of the recently approved orphan drugs include Glaxo's Lexiva (Fosamprenavir) for HIV infection, Genzyme's Fabrazyme (Agalsidase beta) for Fabry

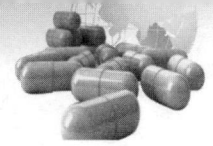

disease, and Novartis's Visudyen (Verteporfin) for age-related macular degeneration.

Australia: The Therapeutic Substances Regulations does not define a rare disease or orphan indication in terms of the number of patients, but rather indicates that it must not be intended for use in more than 2000 patients a year if it is a vaccine or *in vivo* diagnostic. In order to attain the orphan designation, "the application must show why the medicine is an orphan drug". In Australia, orphan drugs are drugs used to treat diseases or conditions affecting fewer than 2,000 individuals at any one time (0.2%).

Canada: Canada has no official "orphan disease" status; however, based on international standards, it could be defined as diseases with a potential patient population numbering between 3,300 (Australian standards) to 22,500 (US definition).

Definition of Orphan Drugs In Asian Countries

India: The need for such an act is thus evident from the initiative by the Indian Pharmacists and the Government to implement Laws, which would strengthen the health infrastructure and provide relief to the numerous rare disease sufferers throughout the country. A group of pharmacologists at a conference held by the Indian Drugs Manufactures Association in 2001 requested the Indian Government to institute the Orphan Drug Act in India.

Taiwan: The official definition of rare disorders is a disease if it is prevalent in 1:10,000 people. On February 9, 2000, Taiwan's Legislative Yuan implemented the Rare Disease and Orphan Drug Act to improve the diagnosis, treatment, and prevention of rare diseases in Taiwan. In particular, the Act aims to provide patients with easier access to pharmaceuticals for the treatment of rare diseases by promoting the supply, manufacturing, and R&D of these products. To carry out the Act, the Department of Health (DOH) established the Committee for the Review and Examination of Rare Diseases and Orphan Drugs. The health standards in Taiwan are among the best in Asia, and the country boasts high life expectancy about 75 years for men and 80 for women.

Korea: For orphan drug designation in Korea, less than 20,000 people in Korea suffer from the disease/condition, or there is no available treatment for the disease/condition in Korea.

In Korea, orphan drugs are supplied to patients by pharmaceutical companies or the Korea Orphan Drug Center. As of October 2002, over 130 orphan drugs have been approved by the KFDA. The orphan drug application process takes around 6–9 months to complete. Some of the recently approved orphan drugs in Korea include Abbott's Kaletra (Lopinavir plus Ritonavir) capsules and solutions for HIV infection and Schering Plough's Bonefos (Disodium Clodronate) solutions and capsules for the treatment of hypercalcemia and osteolysis due to malignancy.

Hong Kong: Hong Kong boasts a small but wealthy population and the country's health care standards are among the highest in Asia. An orphan drug applicant may register their drug under the New Chemical Entity (NCE) registration process, which was established for new, life saving drugs. In this case, the application will be processed immediately and reviewed by the Hong Kong DOH Pharmaceutical Licensing Committee. This Committee only meets four times a year, so applicants should make an effort to submit their application several weeks prior to a Committee meeting to reduce processing time. A second registration process is available for those applicants which cannot meet the NCE application requirements. The second option, registering under the "normal" registration process, takes 6–9 months to complete.

Singapore: Like Hong Kong, Singapore is small but economically advanced, offering a highly developed health care system.

Singapore's Medicines Act regulates pharmaceuticals in the country, specifically mentions orphan drugs, that portion of the law has never been "activated". Therefore, the definition of an orphan drug is not 100% clear in Singapore and companies can encounter difficulty receiving orphan drug designation. The following information will be supportive in making an orphan drug claim.

i. The drug is used in life-threatening conditions and plays a critical role in the management of that condition.

ii. The disease/condition currently affects a very limited number of patients.

iii. A rough estimate of the number of patients affected by the disease/condition should be provided.

If the drug meets the above conditions and is designated as an orphan drug by the Ministry of Health, it will be given top priority during the registration process. To date, reimbursement of orphan drugs in Singapore has been very challenging.

RARE DISEASE FACTS AND STATISTICS

Here are a few statistics and facts to illustrate the breadth of the rare disease challenge in the United States and worldwide.

1. There are approximately 7,000 different types of rare diseases and disorders, with more being discovered each day.

2. 30 million people in the United States are living with rare diseases. This equates to 1 in 10 Americans or 10 percent of the population.

3. It is estimated that 350 million people worldwide suffer from rare diseases.

4. If all of the people with rare diseases lived in one country, it would be the world's third most populous country. In the United States, a condition is considered "rare" if it affects fewer than 200,000 people.

5. About 80 percent of rare diseases are genetic in origin, and thus are present throughout a person's life, even if symptoms do not immediately appear.

6. The prevalence distribution of rare diseases is skewed—80 percent of all rare disease patients are affected by approximately 350 rare diseases.

7. According to the Every Life Foundation for rare diseases, 95 percent of rare diseases lack a single FDA approved treatment.

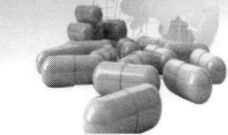

Causes of Rare Diseases

The certain rare diseases that have been named and characterized for decades, investigators still have not determined the cause. For example, although the disease was identified decades ago, no cause is known for Gorham's disease, an extremely rare bone disorder that has been described under more than a dozen different names. Similarly, the Vasculitis Research Consortium, which is part of the NIH-funded Rare Diseases Clinical Research Network, is investigating six forms of vasculitis (a group of rare conditions affecting blood vessels) for which the causes are not known. The causes of rare diseases are mentioned below:

1. Genetic

The majority of rare diseases (approx 80 percent or more) are genetic in origin. Many, if not most are caused by defects in a single gene, for example, alpha 1-antitrypsin deficiency (which may cause serious lung or liver disease). Multiple different mutations in that single gene may result in disease of varying features or severity. Other diseases, such as Fanconi anemia, have several named variants, each caused by a defect in a different gene. In some rare conditions, multiple genes may contribute collectively to manifestations of the disorder.

2. Infectious agents

Rare diseases may be due to infectious causes. Despite their rarity, some infections such as rabies, botulism, and Rocky Mountain spotted fever are relatively well publicized and feared. Some infections are thought to be rare worldwide. In some poor countries most commonly occurring disease are like tuberculosis.

3. Toxic agents

Some rare diseases or conditions result from exposure to natural or manufactured toxic substances, including substances that appear as product contaminant, for examples arsenic and mercury poisoning, mesothelioma (a cancer caused by exposure to asbestos).

4. Other causes

Rare conditions may have a variety of other causes like conditions caused by nutritional deficiencies, e.g. beriberi, which results from thiamine deficiency and is rare in the United States and injuries.

To promote the research and development of orphan drugs by pharmaceutical companies incentives are given by the governments of various countries which are discussed below. For the development and commercialization of new medicines, lot of money and time is involved and moreover, the success rate of new medicines is less. Hence, we cannot expect a pharmaceutical company to work on medicines used for the treatment of rare diseases, since the market for rare diseases is very less. Hence, there is a need for providing incentives in order to encourage pharmaceutical companies which are involved in developing orphan drugs. The following are general encouragement provided by governments of various countries:

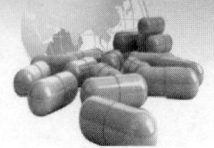

  i. Tax incentives.
 ii. Enhanced patent protection and marketing rights.
iii. Clinical research financial subsidization.
 iv. Creating a government-run enterprise to engage in research and development.

Important Legislations Related to Orphan Drugs in the USA and EU

1. Orphan Drug Act of 1983

It is a law passed in the United States designed to facilitate the development and commercialization of drugs to treat rare diseases, called *orphan drugs*. Orphan drug designation does not indicate that the therapeutic is either safe and effective or legal to manufacture and market in the United States.

Important features of Orphan Drug Act 1983

  i. The companies developing orphan drugs have marketing exclusivity for 7 years.
 ii. The companies may get clinical trial tax incentives.
iii. The companies may have reduced taxes from the federal government.

2. Rare Diseases Act

This legislation amended the Public Health Service Act to establish the Office of Rare Diseases in the USA. It also increased funding for the development of treatments for patients with rare diseases.

3. Regulation (EC) No 141/2000 of the European Union

  i. This legislation lays down a community procedure for the designation of medicinal products as orphan medicinal products.
 ii. It provides incentives for the research, development and placing on the market of designated orphan medicinal products.
iii. It sets up a Committee for Orphan Medicinal Products (COMP) within the Agency.
 iv. Orphan drug status granted by the European Commission gives marketing exclusivity in the EU for 10 years after approval.
  v. In addition to the United States and the European Union, legislation has been implemented by Japan, Singapore, and Australia which have all passed legislation that offers subsidies and other incentives to encourage the development of drugs that treat orphan diseases.

Regulatory Agencies Associated with Orphan Drugs

(a) **FDA Office of Orphan Product Development (OOPD):** The OOPD has following roles:
  i. Evaluates scientific and clinical data submissions from sponsors to identify and designate products as promising for rare disease and to further advance scientific development of such promising medical products.
 ii. It provides incentives for sponsors to develop products for rare diseases.

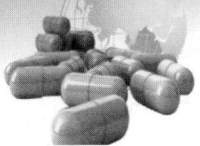

(b) National Organization for Rare Disorders (NORD)

i. It is a NGO based in the USA, involved in providing information, advocacy, research, and patient services to help all patients and families affected by rare diseases.

ii. It was involved in lobbying along with other organizations for passing Orphan Drug Act in the USA.

(c) Committee for Orphan Medicinal Products (COMP)

i. It is one of the scientific committee of EMA that is responsible for reviewing applications from people or companies seeking orphan medicinal product designation.

ii. It is also responsible for advising the European Commission on the establishment and development of a policy on orphan medicinal products in the EU, and assists the Commission in drawing up detailed guidelines and liaising internationally on matters relating to orphan medicinal products.

(d) European Organization for Rare Diseases (EURORDIS): It is an NGO based in Europe, dedicated towards improving quality of life of all people living with rare diseases in Europe.

Orphan drug market exclusivity: The orphan drug marketing followed exclusively in various countries is listed in Table 5.1.

Table 5.1: Orphan drug market exclusivity		
S. No.	*Countries*	*Marketing exclusivity in years*
1.	USA	7 yrs
2.	Europe	10 yrs
3.	Korea	6 yrs
4.	Singapore	10 yrs
5.	Japan	10 yrs
6.	Taiwan	10 yrs

Orphan Drug Policies: The various countries orphan drug policies are illustrated in Table 5.2.

Table 5.2: Orphan drug regulations in different countries	
Country	*Orphan Drug Regulation*
Australia	No orphan drug policy special access scheme (SAS) for unapproved drugs provision for reduction of fees under cost recovery for products used to treat rare but clinically significant conditions for which there is only a limited market

Contd.

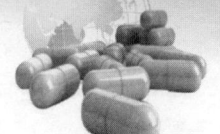

Table 5.2: Orphan drug regulations in different countries *(Contd.)*	
Country	*Orphan Drug Regulation*
Canada	No orphan drug policy
	i. Emergency drug release program/investigational new drugs (EDRP/IND) provides access to unapproved drugs
	ii. SR and ED [scientific research (SR) and experimental development (ED)] tax incentive program would support R and D in the area of orphan drugs
	iii. Provision for reduction of fees for small market drugs under cost recovery
	iv. Process patents granted for biotechnology products
European Union	Development of an orphan drug policy is part of the 1996 work program
	The policy includes:
	i. Designation based on prevalence of disease in the population of less than 0.05% (about 180,000 patients)
	ii. Shared cost program to support research.
Japan	Has orphan drug program
	i. Designation granted based on prevalence of disease in the population of less than 0.05%
	ii. Grant program for R and D for manufacturers and importers of orphan drugs
	iii. Guidance and advice available to industry on both R&D and NDA application procedures
	iv. Tax incentives granted to manufacturers doing R&D on orphan drugs
	v. NDA for orphan drugs are given priority review
UK	No orphan drug policy
	Historically, some government research funds have been made available for the development of drugs for rare diseases
	i. Practitioners can procure unapproved drugs for individual patients based on clinical judgment
	ii. An application under exceptional circumstances can be made when insufficient information on the safety, quality, and/or efficacy of a product.
US	Orphan drug act (January 4, 1983)
	i. Designation granted based on prevalence of disease in the population of less than 200,000 people (approximately 0.1%) or no reasonable expectation of profitability
	ii. Protocol assistance to design research protocols

Contd.

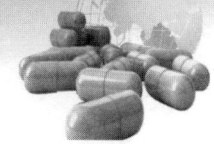

Table: 5.2 Orphan drug regulations in different countries (Contd.)	
Country	*Orphan Drug Regulation*
	iii. Tax credits for clinical research
	iv. Market exclusivity
	v. Funding grants for clinical research to support development
	vi. Penalty for intentionally false statement of orphan status
	vii. Parallel track program and treatment INDs provide access to unapproved drugs
	viii. Process patents granted for biotechnology products accelerated approvals

Big pharmaceutical companies involved in the manufacture of orphan drugs are:

1. Pfizer
2. GlaxoSmithKline
3. Roche
4. Novartis
5. Merck
6. Eli Lilly
7. Johnson and Johnson
8. Bayer
9. Genzyme and Actelion are orphan drug specialist

Significant Results Due to Support of Orphan Drugs

i. Many orphan drugs have been developed to treat rare diseases like Hodgkin's lymphoma, congenital factor XIII deficiency, glioma, multiple myeloma, cystic fibrosis, phenylketonuria, snake venom poisoning, neoplastic meningitis, etc.

ii. Before enactment of ODA in the USA, only 38 drugs were approved to treat orphan diseases. From the passage of the ODA in 1983 until May 2010, the FDA approved 353 orphan drugs and granted orphan designations to 2,116 compounds, which is a significant achievement.

iii. Although the European Medicines Agency grants market access to its 27 member states, medicines only reach the market when each member state decides that its national health system will reimburse for the drug. For example, 35 orphan drugs reached the market in Belgium, 44 in the Netherlands, and 28 in Sweden in 2008. 35 such drugs reached the market in France and 23 in Italy in 2007.

The Orphan Drug Act (ODA) came into effect in 1983 as a solution to meet an unmet need in the industry. Its success is often projected as an example of how innovative regulatory frameworks can be used to develop unviable but necessary solutions. The orphan drug sector has come a long way since the early 1980s. In a recent study, BCC estimated the market size of the sector to be around $85 billion

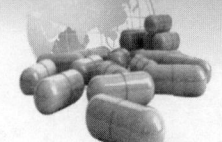

in 2009; this is expected to grow at a compound average growth rate of 6% between 2009 and 2014. ODA provided the biopharma industry a space to grow free of competition from big pharma, and biopharmaceutical companies played a significant role in the development of the orphan drug market. According to the BCC report, biologic orphan drugs accounted for almost 65% of the total orphan drug market in 2009—up from the 60% estimated in 2006.

Although it took almost two decades, big pharma players are now aggressively entering this sector. In 2009, big pharma accounted for 43% of the total orphan drug approvals by the FDA and claimed over 70% of the market share—up from an estimated 53% in 2006. The rising presence of big pharma indicates the importance of ODA in their strategic decisions.

Drying drug pipelines, profit erosions due to generic competition, ever increasing regulatory requirements, and spiralling drug development costs are the key factors driving big pharma's interest in this sector.

As the sustainability of the traditional blockbuster business model wavered, niche busters such as Gleevec instigated tremendous interest in the orphan drug sector. In 2006, there were 19 orphan blockbuster drugs, in 2009 that number was 27. In 2009, 58 orphan drugs generated over $200 million in revenues, although the revenues were not exclusively from orphan indications. The point being emphasized here is that developers are willing to invest in additional clinical trials to establish the effectiveness of their blockbuster drugs in treating rare diseases.

The main attraction of the orphan drug sector is the availability of a market space devoid of competition, which offers freedom in terms of pricing. In addition, rarity of the diseases often justifies small clinical trials that offer substantial bottom-line profitability. Moreover, orphan drugs may get conditional approvals even before the completion of the full clinical trial period.

Unlike standard drugs, orphan drugs do not require mass marketing. Hence, marketing budgets are significantly lower and are targeted to a focused group of specialist physicians and patient advocacy groups. These compelling advantages are driving big pharma investments for developing orphan drug pipelines.

Companies such as Novartis, Eli Lilly, Pfizer, and GlaxoSmithKline (GSK) have invested in active orphan drug development programs. GSK launched a dedicated unit to specialize in orphan drug research in February 2010.

Development of Drug for Rare Disease

The development of any drug is a very complicated process due to the limited patient populations. Typically the disease is less well understood and there are fewer patients to access for testing to prove the drug works.

1. Discovery of Compound

This is the process by which scientists work to discover at the molecular level a compound to affect diseased cells with a certain type of "drug". Based on the biochemistry of the disease, the scientists can either rescreen/repurpose existing drugs or they can develop an entirely new compound.

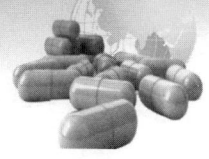

2. Preclinical Research

The proposed compound is refined in the laboratory, usually using cell cultures of some sort. The compound is optimized for safety and efficacy and then further tested, often with animals, to determine whether or not the "drug" is safe enough and has enough promise of efficacy to test on humans.

3. IRB and FDA Approval for Studies in Humans

The researcher packages up all of their lab and animal study data, along with a proposed clinical trial design and applies to both their local Institutional Review Board (IRB) and the FDA for approval for a Clinical Trial. The FDA application is often in the form of a Investigational New Drug (IND) application. Either the IRB and/or the FDA may ask the researcher to provide more data and/or to make changes in the design of the clinical trial. The clinical trial design includes specific criteria for who can participate in the trial, what are being tests, how it is being tested, and very specific "endpoints" that will be monitored determine whether the drug worked or not. The guidelines for clinical trial design and review are established by Congress and enforced by the FDA. Rare diseases place a special burden on the trial designer and regulators due to often somewhat limited knowledge about the natural course of the disease, its biochemistry, the very limited patient populations, and the fact that many of these disease are very aggressive and affect children. The FDA often struggles applying regulations designed for chronic diseases to the quite different rare disease environment.

4. Phase I, II, and III Clinical Trials

Clinical Trials are performed on humans, usually those affected by a particular disease. The purpose of a clinical trial is to prove or disprove a hypothesis.

These trials are very structured with specific inclusion and exclusion criteria as well as very specific endpoints and outcome tests that determine if the hypothesis is correct or not. This criterion is set in advance and is normally not able to be changed during the trial. The Principal Investigator (PI) is in charge of the trial. The PI often wants very close control of the trial, perhaps even by limiting the number of sites to reduce variability and to maintain close tabs on all adverse events , all of which, no matter how small, must be reported to the FDA for review.

Phase I is a safety study—usually performed on a small group of patients.

Phase II is a dosing study—to determine the dosing for the larger efficacy trials. With rare diseases, Phase I and II are often combined into a Phase I/II study.

Phase III tests efficacy—the FDA wants efficacy studied on a large population, but in rare diseases this many only be one or two dozen individuals. With rare diseases, Phases II and III are sometimes combined into a Phase II/III study.

5. New Drug Approval (NDA) Application

With rare diseases, the NDA Application usually comes after Phase III (with chronic condition research it is after Phase IV). The NDA is a very lengthy document covering all aspects of the basic research and clinical trials, including all adverse events. The FDA has a specified period of time to review NDA's and to respond to the application. The guidelines for NDA review and final approval are established by Congress.

6. Post-approval Studies and Final Approval

Phase IV study for rare diseases often comes after market release to continue to study the drug across a broader population while still gathering review data in a structured fashion. Phase IV studies for rare disease may involve the entire eligible patient community making final approval somewhat moot as all patients are already receiving treatment.

PATENTING OF ORPHAN DRUG

The provisions on patent term restoration were part of a larger bill that established a pathway for FDA to approve generic versions of brand name drugs. The goals were to make less expensive versions of brand name drugs more widely available to consumers while still providing incentives for pharmaceutical companies to develop novel drugs. To accomplish the latter objective, the legislation created two new "data exclusivity" rules. The first exclusivity rule provides that truly innovative drugs—new chemical entities (also called new molecular entities)—receive a 5-year period of data exclusivity, during which the sponsor of a generic drug must submit a full New Drug Application that relies on its own preclinical and clinical data. At the end of 5 years, the applicant can submit an ANDA that need only show that its product is the same as, and bioequivalent to, the innovator's product. A generic product is the same as the innovator product if it has the same active ingredient, route of administration, dosage form, and strength. The law permits differences in these characteristics, with prior agency approval, if no clinical data are needed to establish the safety or effectiveness of the generic product. Generally, a generic drug is bioequivalent to the innovator product if there is not a significant difference in the rate and extent of absorption of the drug when administered at the same molar dose of the therapeutic ingredient under similar experimental conditions. The second exclusivity rule provides that other applications for approval that are supported by clinical data (e.g. those involving new formulations of the drug) receive 3 years of exclusivity. Again, during the period of exclusivity, generic versions can be approved only if sponsors provide their own clinical data on safety and efficacy.

Ultraorphan Drugs

Ultraorphan drug development is still challenging. However, some of the emerging business models may change the industry outlook on ultraorphan drugs. The inventors and adapters of these innovative business models include not-for-profit as well as for-profit companies, pharmacies, and patient-support groups.

While the for-profit business model based on high-prices has become the norm of the sector, novel approaches are being adopted in the emerging ones. For instance, the Institute for One World Health, a not-for-profit company focusing exclusively on neglected diseases, works on a hybrid business model combining philanthropic

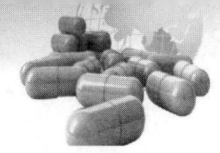

funding with the revenues from commercial activities such as partnership projects and intellectual property licensing.

Another model is patient-support groups as investors. A typical example is the Cystic Fibrosis Foundation Therapeutics, which is promoting cystic fibrosis drug development by acting as a virtual company based on a venture philanthropy business model.

Specialty pharmacies dedicated exclusively to ultraorphan drugs are also emerging, which is proving to be beneficial for patients as well as companies. While the patients receive a full package of services that include safe and timely delivery, payment, reimbursement, and financial assistance, the companies benefit by improved patient access that assists in patient monitoring and price designing.

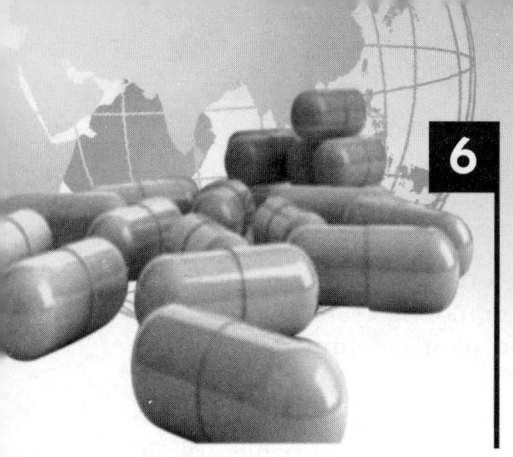

6 Drug Regulatory Approval Process for Advanced Countries

The new drug approval process for the European countries involves two stages:
 (a) First stage involves clinical research.
 (b) Second stage involves regulatory approval of the medicinal product.

After clinical studies when the product has been completed, an application is given to the competent authority to obtain approval for the product. The competent authority reviews the application and permits marketing authorization for the product, if it is effective and safe and its desirable effects overweigh its adverse affects for human beings.

Even after the approval of new drug, government should monitor its safety due to some side effects, after using it on large population. The interactions with other drugs, which were not assessed in a pre-marketing research trial and its adverse effects (in particular populations), should also be monitored. The regulatory procedures used by the EU countries are detailed below:

Drug Regulatory Approval Process in Europe

In European Union (EU), the medical products were approved for marketing at the National level initially. The mutual recognition procedure was introduced in 1983 and a single national review in case of pharmaceutical/medicinal product for marketing authorizations in all the EU's countries was made feasible. The primary aim of this procedure was to create a united standard for product review among national regulatory authorities. In 1987, for high-technology or biologically derived products, the concertation procedure was established by directive 87/22, in which product assessment should be completed by Committee for Proprietary Medicinal Products (CPMP) besides the normal national regulatory review. Further, in 1993, by council regulation (EEC) 2309/93, the concertation procedure was replaced with centralized procedure, by which all the high-tech and biologically derived product was reviewed and granted EU's wide marketing authorization by the EU's CPMP. In all the European procedures, the regulatory approval process must be completed within 210 days or earlier.

Similarly, the drug approval process in the European countries is also accomplished in two phases: Clinical trial and marketing authorization. A clinical

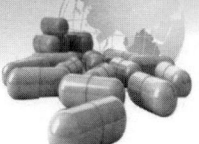

trial application (CTA) is filed to the competent authority of the state to conduct the clinical trial within EU. The competent authority of that member state evaluates the application. The clinical trials are conducted only after the approval. The purpose and phases of clinical trials are similar as specified in FDA drug approval process. Figure 6.1 represents the clinical trial authorization process in EU.

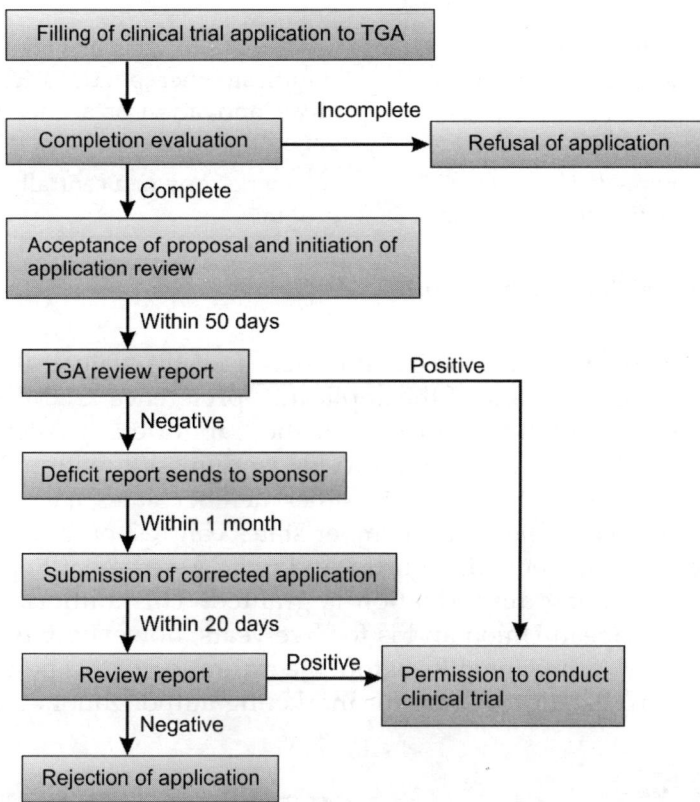

Fig. 6.1: Clinical trial authorization process in Europe

After completing of all three phases of clinical trial, marketing authorization application is filed including all animal and human data, its analyses, as well as pharmacokinetics, manufacturing and proposed labeling. In the EU's countries, the companies have a choice of following regulatory procedures:

• Centralized procedure—for eligible products (Table 6.1)
• Decentralized procedure, national procedure, mutual recognition procedure—for other products.

Centralized Procedure

Products eligible for the centralized procedure: The centralized procedure is used by the European Medicines Agency (EMA). This procedure involves a single application, and when approved, it is valid in all member states of the European Union.

Table 6.1: Centralized procedure for eligible products	
Mandatory	*Optional*
Human medicines for the treatment of HIV/AIDS, cancer, diabetes, neurodegenerative diseases, autoimmune and other immune dysfunctions, and viral diseases	Other new active substances not authorized in the European community before May 20, 2004
Medicines derived from biotechnology processes, such as genetic engineering	Medicinal products that contribute significant therapeutic, scientific, or technical innovation or are in the interest of patient health
Advanced therapy medicines such as gene therapy, somatic cell therapy, or tissue engineered medicines	A generic copy of a centrally authorized product
Officially designated "orphan medicines"	

The Committee for Human Medicinal Products (CHMP) evaluate the applications received by the EMEA. In view of the applicant's preference, CHMP contracts out assessment work in one of the member states (the "rapporteur"). After the complete assessment, the CHMP deliver opinion to EU Commission within 210 days. The EU Commission requests comments from other member states, if a positive opinion from CHMP is received. The other member states can respond in about 28 days. When a licence is recommended, a European Public Assessment Report (EPAR) is produced and marketing authorization is granted. This authorization is valid throughout the European Union and is for five years, however, the extension can be applied to the EMA three months before the expiration of this period. Figure 6.2 represents the centralized procedure for marketing authorization.

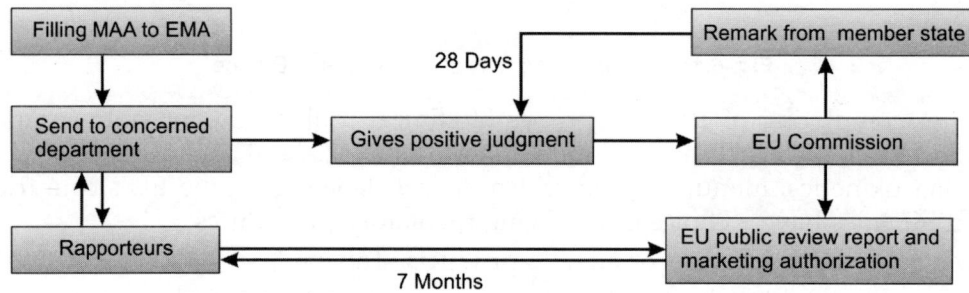

Fig. 6.2: EU centralized procedure for marketing authorization

EMA—European medicines agency; MAA—marketing authorization application

Decentralized Procedure

In order to obtain marketing authorizations in several member states, the centralized procedure is not mandatory; in such case the decentralized procedure is to be used. An application is submitted to competent authorities of each of the member states,

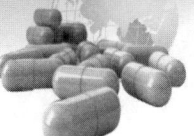

where a marketing authorization is to be sought. The information like quality, efficacy, safety, administrative information shall be submitted and a list of all Concerned Member States (CMSs) and one member state to act as Reference Member State (RMS). A draft assessment report on the medicinal product is prepared and the CMSs and the RMS validate the application within a time frame of 14 days. The RMS prepare draft summary of product characteristics, labeling and package leaflet within 120 days. This report can be approved within 90 days. However, if a medicinal product is supposed to cause potential serious risk to public health, CMS(s) will inform to other CMS, RMS and applicant and further decision in this regard is taken within 30 days. Within 60 days of the communication of the points of disagreement, all member states reach to an agreement on the action to be taken (Fig. 6.3). After reaching to an

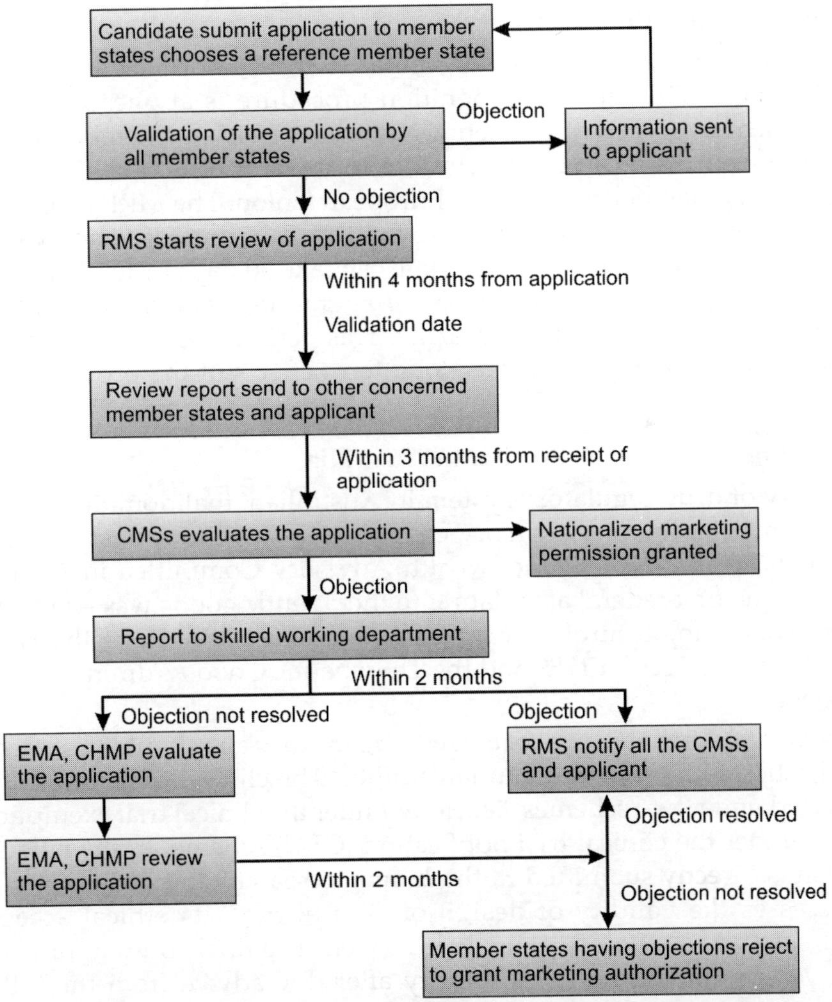

```
Candidate submit application to member
states chooses a reference member state
                 │
                 ▼                          Objection
Validation of the application by ─────────────────────▶  Information sent
all member states                                        to applicant
                 │
                 ▼ No objection
RMS starts review of application
                 │
                 │ Within 4 months from application
                 │
                 │ Validation date
                 ▼
Review report send to other concerned
member states and applicant
                 │
                 │ Within 3 months from receipt of
                 │ application
                 ▼
CMSs evaluates the application ──────────▶  Nationalized marketing
                 │                          permission granted
                 ▼ Objection
Report to skilled working department
                 │
                 │ Within 2 months
        ┌────────┴────────────────────────────┐
        ▼ Objection not resolved      Objection ▼
EMA, CHMP evaluate                    RMS notify all the CMSs
the application                       and applicant
        │                                      ▲
        ▼                              Objection resolved
EMA, CHMP review
the application ──── Within 2 months ──┘
                                       Objection not resolved
                                               ▼
                              Member states having objections reject
                              to grant marketing authorization
```

Fig. 6.3: EU decentralized procedure for marketing authorization

CMS(s)—Concerned member state(s); RMS—reference member state; CHMP—committee for human medicinal products; EMA—European medicine agency

agreement of the member states, the RMS records the agreement and informs to the applicant. However, if the member states could not reach an agreement, then CHMP intervenes and take a final decision keeping in view of the written or oral explanations of the applicant. Figure 6.3 represents the decentralized procedure for marketing authorization in EU.

Human Medicinal Products

National Procedure

This type of authorization is granted on country-by-country basis by the competent authorities, in each member state. Products only intended for one market and not obliged to use the centralized procedure.

Mutual Recognition Procedure

The mutual recognition procedure is similar to the decentralized procedure with some differences. The mutual recognition procedure is applicable to medicinal products which have received marketing authorization in any member state whereas the decentralized procedure is applicable to those products which were never approved in any member states of the European Union. The MRP is used to obtain marketing authorizations in various several member states. The evaluation of application by the Reference Member State can take 90 days instead of 120 days (as is the case with decentralized procedure). After granting of marketing authorization, the product may be placed on the market. This period is also known as Phase IV where new uses or new populations, long-term effects of the product, etc. can be investigated.

Drug Regulatory Approval Process in Australia

In the history of drug regulatory system in Australian, thalidomide disaster was a key factor. In 1948, the first advisory committee to review drugs was set up and further in 1964, the first Commonwealth Advisory Committee in Australia was established. The first federal act relating to therapeutic goods was enacted in 1965. In response of lacking control over locally manufactured products, the Therapeutic Goods Act was changed in 1989 and the Therapeutic Goods Administration (TGA) was created.

Any person seeking approval of a new drug in Australia should first file a clinical trial application for conducting human studies. The clinical trials in Australia can be conducted under two schemes, i.e. either under the clinical trial exemption (CTX) scheme or under the clinical trial notification (CTN) scheme. In the latter scheme, application is directly submitted to the human research ethics committee (HREC) which assesses the validity of design of clinical trial, its ethical acceptability, approval, safety and efficacy of the drug as well. The final consent for conducting trial is given by the approving authority after due advice from the HREC. The commencement of clinical trial takes place only after the due notification to the TGA and the appropriate notification fee to be paid. In CTX scheme, an application to conduct clinical trials is submitted to the TGA for evaluation and comment. The

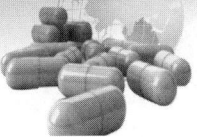

clinical trials can be conducted (under the CTX application) without further assessment by the TGA and the conduct of each trial should be notified to the TGA. An application is submitted to TGA to register the drug in Australian Register of Therapeutic Goods (ARTG) after the completion of clinical trials. The application consists of data to support the quality, safety and efficacy of the product for its intended use. The application is assessed (on an administrative level) to make sure for compliance with basic guidelines and further evaluated by different sections and advice can also be sought on key issues to take final decision. A company can make comments on the evaluation report, if necessary. A delegate (decision-maker) within the TGA after due advice of the ADEC, take a decision to approve or reject the product. The Australian Drug Evaluation Committee (ADEC) usually gives advice for new medicines. When the drug is approved and distributed in the market the drug, it is considered to be in Phase IV trials. In this phase, new uses or new populations, long-term effects, etc. can be explored.

Drug Approval Process in Turkey

In Turkey, new drugs are granted marketing authorization after reviewing their safety, efficacy and quality. The General Directorate of Pharmaceuticals and Pharmacy (ÝEGM) is charged with the marketing authorization process, and is the principal national authority for approval, pricing, legal classification and inspection of drugs. The General Directorate is supported by scientific committees in conducting medical, pharmaceutical and clinical evaluations of products proposed for approval. Committees evaluate documents submitted by pharmaceutical manufacturers, and their decisions provide the basis for marketing authorization and licensure. The application is initially reviewed by the Advisory Committee for Registration of human medicinal products, usually taking 3 to 4 months. The third step in the marketing authorization process involves setting the product price, which is the responsibility of ÝEGM pricing branch. Thus, pricing is a part of the regulatory approval process. The price is set using an external reference price chart. The pricing procedure usually takes 3 to 6 months. After completion of pricing negotiations, the committee reviews the application for bioequivalence (for generic products) and bioavailability (for original products).

For alignment with the European Union regulations, the registration regulation of human medicinal products requires following the common technical document (CTD) guidelines for preparing the marketing authorization application file.

The General Directorate of Pharmaceuticals and Pharmacy was the sole authority charged with granting marketing authorization and selling permits for, and pricing, classifying and reviewing drugs in Turkey.

According to the registration regulation of human medicinal products, the ministry conducts a preliminary review to evaluate whether the marketing authorization application file is complete and free from any omissions in terms of the requisite data and documents which must be submitted, depending on the type of application and applicable requirements laid down in the registration regulation of human medicinal products. The ministry completes the administrative review and notifies its outcome to the applicant within 30 (thirty) days after receipt of the application file at the ministry. In the event that deficiencies are identified, the applicant has 30 (thirty) days to address such deficiencies. The second preliminary review, conducted after omissions have been addressed and resubmitted to the Ministry, is completed also within one month.

In the event that ministry's preliminary review finds the applicant to be lacking the requisite qualifications prescribed in the Registration Regulation of Human Medicinal Products, or the file submitted for second preliminary review is again found to be marred by omissions, the application is rejected and returned to the applicant.

According to the Registration Regulation of Human Medicinal Products, the Ministry must complete its regulatory review of the file within 210 (two hundred and ten) days, provided the application file is free from any omissions and has cleared through the preliminary review according to the Registration Regulation of Human Medicinal Products. However, the clock stops for the duration of any extraordinary circumstances or until the applicant submits any data or documents requested by the ministry, which do not count toward the 210 days timeframe.

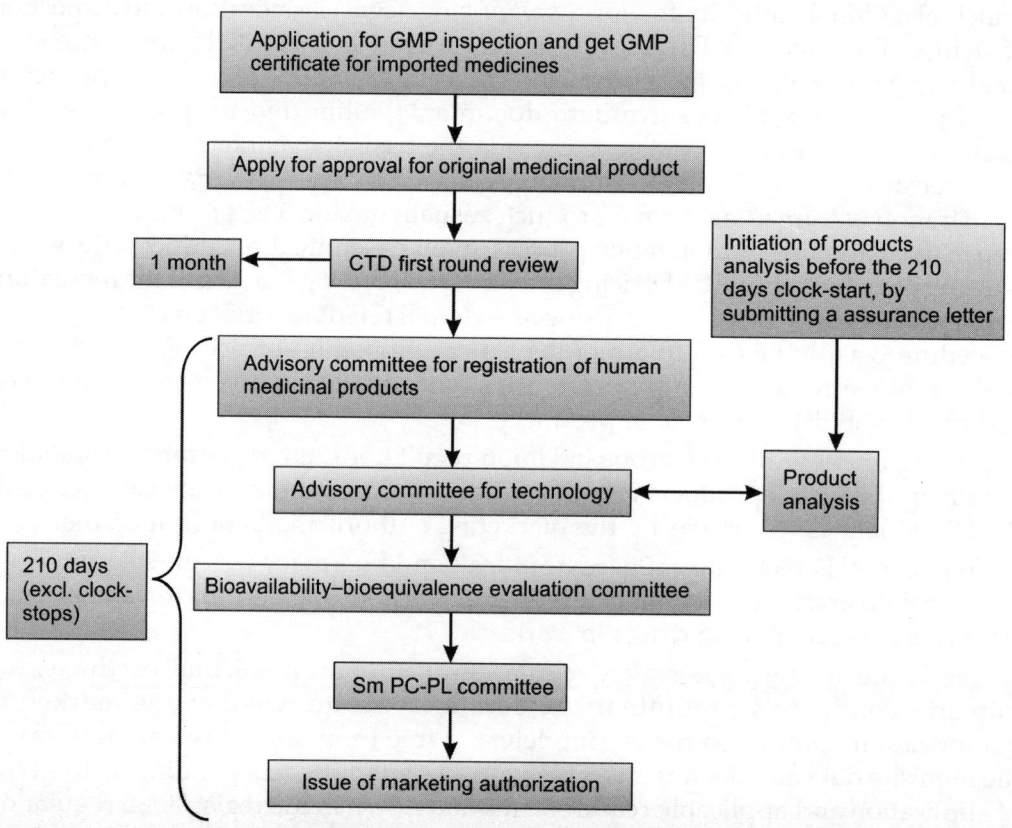

Fig. 6.4: Overview of the regulatory approval procedure in Turkey

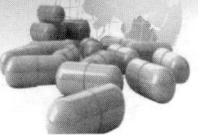

The registration regulation of human medicinal products lists the following product-related criteria for granting marketing authorization to a human medicinal product: the efficacy of the product has been proven under its intended conditions of use, the safety of the product has been proven, and the product has the appropriate technical and pharmaceutical characteristics. The ministry may, however, waive some of these criteria taking account of pharmacoeconomic data, when public health considerations warrant it. Marketing authorization is granted to products which, according to data and documents submitted to and reviewed and analyzed by the ministry, fulfill the requirements of the registration regulation of human medicinal products.

Before offering a product for sale for the first time after receipt of marketing authorization, product samples representative of the final commercial product must be submitted to the ministry to obtain a "selling permit." The ministry reviews the samples for conformity of the package leaflet, package and label information, and price, and grants a selling permit if the product meets the requirements. In view of the above procedural details, the regulatory approval procedure in Turkey is outlined in Fig. 6.4.

DRUG REGULATORY APPROVAL PROCESS FOR CANADA

Pharmaceutical drugs are mostly synthetic products made from chemicals. They are meant to improve the health and well-being of patients by helping to prevent and treat disease, reduce pain and suffering, extend and save lives. Some higher-risk drugs, such as those used to treat diseases, require a prescription from a physician. Other lower-risk drugs, such as cough syrup and antacids, are sold without a prescription and are readily available to the public.

Pharmaceutical drugs play an important role in Canada's health care system and economy. With an aging population, the role of pharmaceutical drugs is expected to grow as researchers come up with new drug therapies to replace earlier treatments or provide new options where no treatment existed before. Canadians who purchase and consume pharmaceuticals authorized for sale in Canada rely on the government and industry to monitor the safety of these products. Health Canada has a responsibility to help protect the public against undue health and safety risks from the use of pharmaceutical drugs.

Health Canada, through the *Food and Drugs Act*, regulates the safety, efficacy, and quality of all pharmaceutical drugs for use by humans in Canada before and after the products enter the Canadian marketplace. The Department does this through a combination of scientific review, monitoring, compliance, and enforcement activities. It aims to ensure that the public has timely access to safe and effective pharmaceutical drugs and that those who need to know of safety concerns are informed.

The Food and Drugs Act (the Act) Defines "Drug"

Any substance or mixture of substances manufactured, sold or represented for use in:

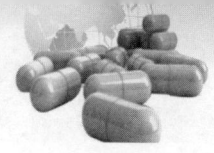

(a) The diagnosis, treatment, mitigation or prevention of a disease, disorder or abnormal physical state, or its symptoms, in human beings or animals,

(b) Restoring, correcting or modifying organic functions in human beings or animals, or

(c) Disinfection in premises in which food is manufactured, prepared or kept.

Health Canada categorizes drugs for human use as prescription drugs, non-prescription drugs, radiopharmaceuticals and biologics.

All regulatory and enforcement activities, and most policy activities, associated with pharmaceuticals are conducted within the Health Products and Food Branch (HPFB) of Health Canada. Directorates within HPFB include one each for food and veterinary drugs and four for drugs, namely:

  i. Therapeutic products directorate (TPD)
  ii. Biologics and genetic therapies directorate (BGTD),
  iii. HPFB inspectorate—compliance and enforcement
  iv. Marketed health products directorate (MHPD),
  v. Natural health products directorate (NHPD), and
  vi. Veterinary drugs directorate (VDD)

Therapeutic Products Directorate

Health Canada's Therapeutic Products Directorate (TPD) is the national authority that regulates evaluates and monitors the safety, efficacy, and quality of therapeutic and diagnostic products available to Canadians. These products include drugs, medical devices, disinfectants and sanitizers with disinfectant claims. Similar to CDER in the US FDA.

Biologics and Genetic Therapies Directorate (BGTD)

Responsible for evaluating the safety, effectiveness and quality of biological and radiopharmaceutical drugs, as well as blood and blood products, viral and bacterial vaccines, genetic therapeutic products, tissues, organs and xenografts. Similar to CBER in the US FDA.

HPFB Inspectorate—Compliance and Enforcement

Responsible for delivery of inspections and investigations and for most establishment licensing and related laboratory analysis functions.

Marketed Health Products Directorate (MHPD)

Responsible for post-market assessment and surveillance of pharmaceutical and biological drugs, medical devices, natural health products, radiopharmaceuticals.

Natural Health Products Directorate (NHPD)

Responsible for ensuring that Canadians have ready access to health products that are safe, effective, and high quality by maintaining proper labeling and implementing regulatory framework which supports freedom of choice and cultural diversity.

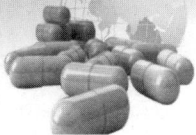

Veterinary Drugs Directorate (VDD)

Ensures the safety of foods such as milk, meat, eggs, fish and honey from animals treated with veterinary drugs, and that veterinary drugs sold in Canada are safe and effective for animals.

The common types of submission in Canada are mentioned below:

(a) NDS: New drug submission. It is similar to NDA in the US. Typically require preclinical, clinical, chemistry and manufacturing data.

(b) ANDS: Abbreviated new drug submission (generics). It is similar to ANDA in the US. Typically required bioequivalence and/or pharmaceutical equivalence data.

(c) SNDS: Supplement to new drug submission. It is similar to SNDA in the US.

Overview of Drug Regulatory Approval Process in Canada (Fig. 6.5)

Pre-market

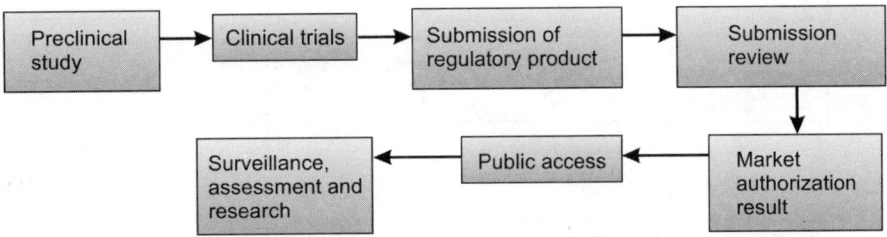

Fig. 6.5: Drug regulatory process in Canada

Following steps are followed for the drug approval process:

1. Clinical Trials of New Drugs

Clinical trials are conducted in human subjects to test the safety and efficacy of newly developed drugs that have shown positive results in preclinical investigation. Testing in humans is conducted in three or four phases:

1. Phase I: Involves a small number of healthy subjects to test the toxicity, absorption, distribution and metabolism of the drug.

2. Phase II: Involves trials with a larger set of individuals suffering from the condition for which the drug was developed, to test efficacy and safety.

3. Phase III: Involves a greater number of people also with the condition in question, to test the drug's performance in relation to a placebo and/or standard therapy.

4. Phase IV: Involves all studies conducted after a drug has received approval that were not considered necessary for approval but are often important for optimizing the drug's use, also referred to as post-market or post-approval studies.

These trials are subject to the clinical trial regulations under part C, division 5 of the Food and Drug Regulations (the Regulations) which seek to ensure: The safety of the participants; the integrity of the study; the validity of the data; and strict controls over the use of an unapproved drug. Authorization to conduct phase I, II, or III clinical trials must be obtained from Health Canada before starting the investigation. Phase IV clinical trials do not require authorization.

2. Regulatory process for drugs approvals in Canada (Fig. 6.6)

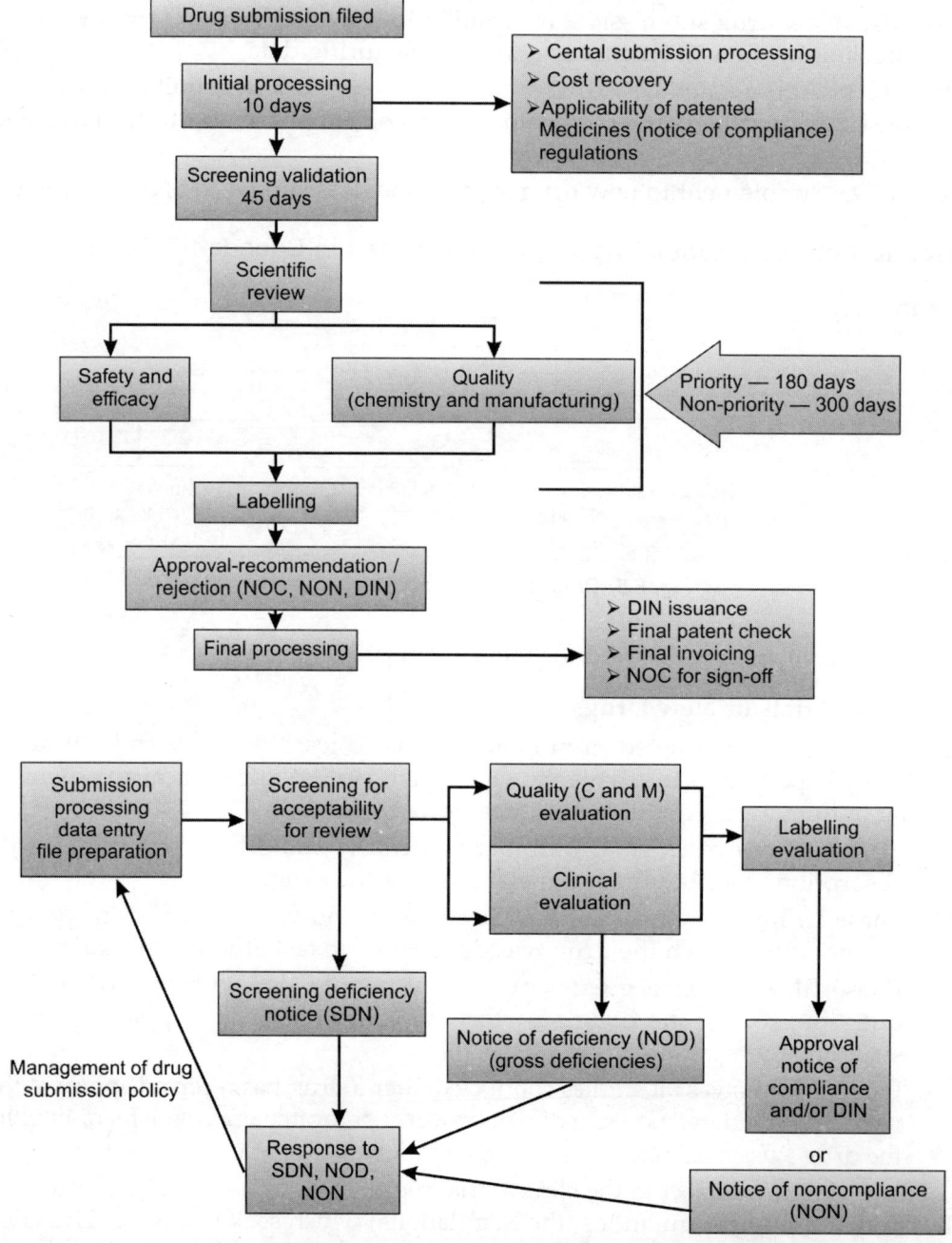

Fig. 6.6: Regulatory process for drugs approvals in Canada

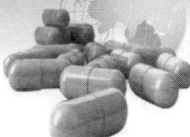

3. New drug approval process involved the below mentioned steps:

(a) *Pre-submission meeting:* Once the developer and/or manufacturer of a new investigational drug is confident that it has produced a compound that can successfully gain Health Canada's approval, a pre-submission meeting is encouraged by TPD, but is not essential. This meeting can be beneficial to the drug sponsor as well as Health Canada as it alerts the regulator to upcoming submissions and allows the sponsor an opportunity to optimize their submission package.

(b) *Submission filing:* This is the first step in the drug approval process. Submission filing involves submitting to TPD a new drug submission, or NDS. The NDS must contain information that: describes the drug; asserts its quality; summarizes the investigational studies and clinical trials pertaining to the drug including adverse reactions observed during clinical trials; and finally, includes raw data from preclinical studies.

(c) *Screening:* When TPD receives an NDS, it first screens the package to ensure that the submission is complete and in the proper format. Health Canada aims to meet a target of 45 calendar days for screening NDSs. Upon a successful screening, the submission proceeds to the technical review. If, however, deficiencies are identified in the submission filing, the sponsor is sent a screening deficiency notice to which it has 45 calendar days to respond and address the noted deficiencies. Unsuccessful candidates are sent a screening rejection letter.

(d) *Technical review:* Upon successful completion of the screening process, the submission passes to the technical review component. TPD has established a target of 300 days for this phase of the drug approval process. Evaluation of the submission involves a detailed review of all the material submitted in the filing in order to produce a comprehensive analysis of the quality, safety and efficacy of the candidate drug and ensures that the risks associated with taking the drug do not outweigh the benefits. Clinical trial data is central to determine the safety/efficacy profile for a candidate drug. At any point during the review TPD can request clarification, re-evaluation or expansion of the submitted material.

Possible outcomes of the technical review are:

i. A notice of deficiency if the submission is incomplete, at which point the review process stops but can resume if the deficiencies are addressed;

ii. A notice of deficiency—withdrawal letter if the applicant does not satisfactorily address deficiencies;

iii. A notice of non-compliance if TPD finds that the submission is incomplete or deficient which lists all deficient or incomplete aspects of the submission, to which the applicant can respond;

iv. A notice of non-compliance—withdrawal letter if the applicant does not respond or if the response is unacceptable at which time the submission will be considered withdrawn;

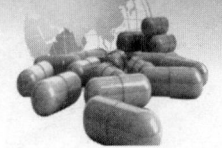

v. A notice of compliance (NOC) which certifies that the drug complies with all requirements of the Act and its regulations. At this time a drug identification number (DIN), an eight digit number, is also issued which authorizes the drug to be marketed in Canada; or,

vi. A notice of decision and a summary basis of decision for each approved drug outlining its risk-benefit analysis which are posted on Health Canada's website.

When TPD issues a NOC for a new drug, the approval extends only as far as the specifics for which the manufacturer initially requested approval. The dosing information, route of administration, labeling, formulation, method of manufacture and indications for use are specified in the NOC and any deviation from these parameters requires a new approval, in which case the manufacturer must file a supplemental new drug submission.

Health Canada also provides two options for expedited review of drugs for serious and life-threatening conditions. First, priority review of a submission may be granted for drugs that are intended for the treatment, prevention or diagnosis of serious, life-threatening or severely debilitating illnesses or conditions for which there is either no product currently marketed in Canada or the new product represents a significant increase in efficacy and/or significant decrease in risk such that the overall risk-benefit profile is better than that of existing therapies. Priority reviews are subject to the same requirements as NDSs, including clinical trial data, but are processed more quickly, whereby the target for screening is reduced to 25 days and the target for the review is 180 days.

The second process for expedited review allows for a reduced threshold of evidence than that required under the NDS process, that is, that the amount of clinical trial evidence may be reduced. Under this category of drug review Health Canada can issue a NOC with conditions (NOC/c) which requires that the manufacturer continue to collect data on the drug's safety and effectiveness, essentially supplementing the clinical trial evidence base to bring it up to the standards required for NDSs.

Similar to priority review, the NOC/c process can be applied to drugs for serious and life-threatening conditions where there is either no product currently marketed in Canada or the new product represents a significant increase in efficacy and/or significant decrease in risk such that the overall risk-benefit profile is better than that of existing therapies. This process allows for a screening target of 25 days and a review target of 200 days.

There is the possibility that new drugs may be approved by Health Canada when the safety, efficacy and quality data on them is limited. Under extraordinary circumstances a drug may be given market authorization with less information from clinical trials than would normally be permitted. These circumstances include emergencies such as exposure to a chemical, biological, radiological or nuclear substance which requires action to treat or prevent the resulting condition. The nature of these circumstances makes it impossible to design and conduct controlled clinical trials to first test the new drug. Therefore, Health Canada's extraordinary

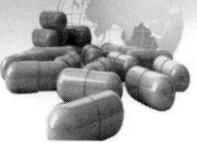

use new drug policy allows approval of these drugs with a little or no clinical trial data.

4. Drug Approval within Health Canada's Biologics and Genetic Therapies Directorate

The approval of biologics, radiopharmaceuticals and genetic therapies is carried out within the Biologics and Genetic Therapies Directorate (BGTD) of HPFB and the process is similar to that for new drugs within TPD, with some differences due to the unique nature of these products. Examples of products regulated by BGTD include cells, tissues and organs (for transplant), vaccines, blood and blood products, gene therapies, and radioactive pharmaceuticals, or radiopharmaceuticals.

Before a biologic can be considered for approval, sufficient scientific evidence must be collected to show that it is safe, efficacious and of suitable quality, as is the case with other drug submissions. Biologics differ from other drugs for human use, however, in that they must include more detailed chemistry and manufacturing information than is required for other drug submissions. Additional information is required for these products in order to ensure their purity and quality because they are more susceptible than other classes of drugs to contamination and variation from one production batch to the next.

As with other classes of drugs described above, biologics and genetic therapies are granted NOCs and DINs once approved by BGTD. However, marketing of these drugs differs from the other drug categories as mentioned below:

Biological drug review also includes:

On-site evaluations

Assessment of the production process and facility for a specific product which ensures that the manufacturing process conforms to information described in the submission.

Additional Good Manufacturing Practices (GMP)

Special considerations and issues pertinent to manufacturing and control of biological drugs, blood and blood components.

Lot-release

Laboratory work on samples received from drug companies to confirm potency, purity and safety. Only high risk products are tested (new products and vaccines).

Generic Drug Approval Process in Canada (ANDS)

Food and Drugs Act and Regulations amended in 1995, allows for a generic manufacturer to file an ANDS, establishment of bioequivalence by requiring a Canadian Reference Product (CRP) same route of administration as CRP, same conditions of use as the CRP ensuring safety, efficacy and high quality. **Canada** defines generic drug as:

A generic drug is a copy of a brand name product, known as the 'reference product'. Generic drugs contain the same medicinal ingredients as the brand name

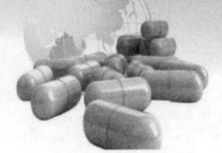

drug, and are considered bioequivalent to the reference product. There may be many generic versions of the same reference product.

The quality standards for brand name drugs and generic drugs are the same. The ingredients, manufacturing processes and facilities for all drugs must meet the federal guidelines for good manufacturing practices. As well, all drug manufacturers must perform a series of tests, both during and after production, to show that every drug batch made meets the requirements for that product. The generic drug must contain the same amount of medicinal ingredient as the brand name reference product. However, non-medicinal ingredients, like fillers and ingredients that color the drug may be different from those of the brand name product. The generic manufacturer must provide studies showing that the different non-medicinal ingredients have not changed the quality, safety or effectiveness of the generic drug. To prove that their products are safe and effective, generic drug manufacturers must demonstrate that the generic drug performs similarly to the brand name drug. The studies that compare the generic drug with the brand name drug are called "comparative bioavailability" studies. In these studies, the level of a medicinal ingredient in the blood of healthy human volunteers is measured. During the studies, each volunteer gets the brand name drug and the new generic drug. The generic drug must show that it delivers the same amount of medicinal ingredient at the same rate as the brand name drug.

Canadian reference drug product refers to:

(a) "A drug in respect of which a notice of compliance is issued pursuant to section C.08.004 and which is marketed in Canada by the innovator of the drug,

(b) A drug, acceptable to the Minister, that can be used for the purpose of demonstrating bioequivalence on the basis of pharmaceutical and, where applicable, bioavailability characteristics, where a drug in respect of which a notice of compliance has been issued pursuant to section C.08.004 cannot be used for that purpose because it is no longer marketed in Canada, or

(c) A drug, acceptable to the Minister, that can be used for the purpose of demonstrating bioequivalence on the basis of pharmaceutical and, where applicable, bioavailability characteristics, in comparison to a drug referred to in paragraph a".

Generic Approval Process in Canada (Fig. 6.7)

Upon receipt of the ANDS, the TPD will undertake a screening process to ensure it is complete and in the appropriate format. This is an administrative review and does not include any technical review of the information. The TPD targets 45 calendar days to complete the screening of an ANDS. Once the screening is complete and accepted, the submission enters the queue for technical review.

If the screening process identifies deficiencies in the ANDS, the sponsor will receive a "screening deficiency notice", and has 45 calendar days to respond and resolve any identified deficiencies. Nowadays industries are getting clarification in form of "Clarifax".

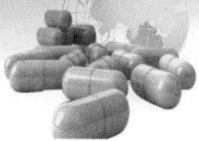

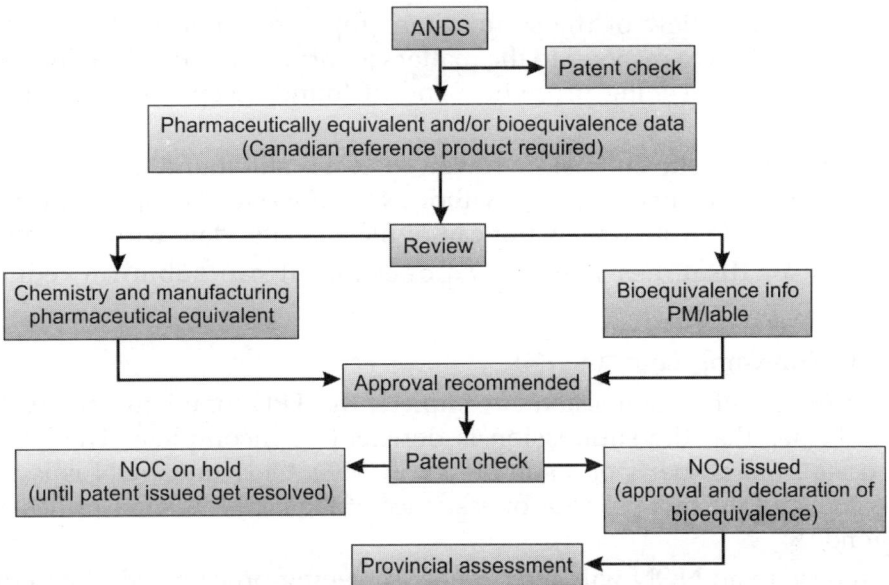

Fig. 6.7: Generic approval process in Canada

Once an ANDS for a generic product passes the screening process and is accepted for review, the TPD has a target of 300 calendar days to complete its evaluation.

If TPD is not able to commence the review of a submission prior to its performance target date, the sponsor will receive an Update Notice, which provides an opportunity for the sponsor to update the file with additional information. The sponsor has 30 days to decide and then notify the TPD if it will submit additional information. The sponsor then has a further 60 days to update its submission.

During the review of a submission, a sponsor can receive a variety of different types of letters requesting additional information.

Clarifax (Clarification request)

A clarifax is a request to expand, clarify or re-analyze existing data. A sponsor has 15 calendar days to respond to a clarifax. If the sponsor is able to meet the timeframe for response, the review will continue uninterrupted. The TPD has no limit on the number of clarifaxes that it may issue in relation to a submission.

Notice of Deficiency (NOD)

If there are significant deficiencies or omissions in a submission that preclude the continuation of the review, the TPD will send an NOD. The NOD will list all deficiencies in the file that has been reviewed to date. The review of all aspects of the submission may not necessarily be complete when the NOD is issued. For example, the clinical review may be complete but the chemistry, manufacturing and controls (CMC) review may not have started. Only one NOD will be issued per submission. Review of the submission stops on issuance of an NOD. The sponsor has 90 days to respond to the matters identified in the NOD. The response goes through the screening procedure and, if found acceptable, it re-enters the review queue.

When the response to an NOD is reviewed, if it is still found to be deficient, the TPD will issue a notice of deficiency–withdrawal (NOD/w). The sponsor is required to withdraw the file from review but can re-file at a later date without prejudice.

If a sponsor disagrees with TPD's decision, it can submit a request for reconsideration.

Notice of Non-compliance (NON)

After the review of a submission is complete, the TPD may issue an NON. This letter indicates that the submission is deficient or incomplete. The NON lists deficiencies from all parts of a submission (CMC). Only one NON is issued per submission, and the review stops on issuance of the NON. A sponsor has 90 days to respond.

A response to an NON will enter a new screening process and, if accepted for review, it will re-enter the queue. If a response to an NON contains unsolicited information or is found to be deficient during screening, the response will be rejected and the submission withdrawn from further review. If a sponsor fails to respond to an NON on time, or if the response is unacceptable, the TPD will issue a notice of

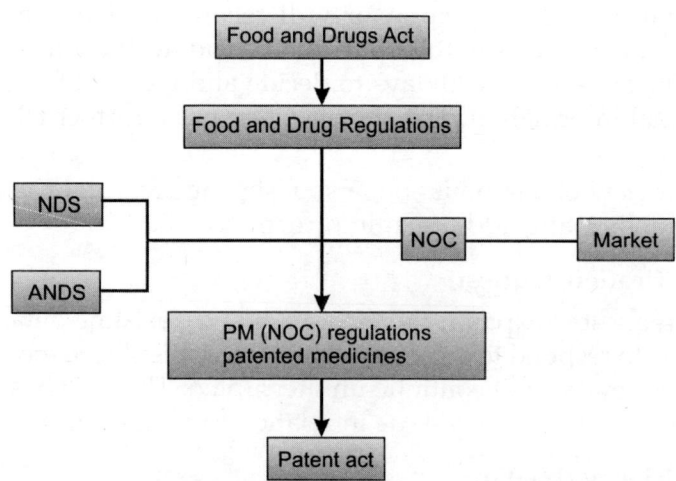

Fig. 6.8: Regulatory scheme in Canada

non-compliance–withdrawal (NON/w).

Figure 6.8 represents the regulatory scheme in Canada.

Role of TPD in improving the efficiency of the drug review process

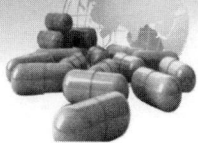

The TPD has been and continues to be committed to ensure the drug review process is as efficient as possible. To do this, the TPD has implemented and is pursuing several initiatives to streamline the process including:

i. Use of electronic drug submission templates;

ii. Participating in the development and implementation of internationally agreed upon products such as technical guidance, a common format and content standard for drug submissions, and standards for the electronic exchange of information;

iii. Implementing and strengthening a team approach to product reviews;

iv. Upgrading and expanding information technology capabilities;

v. Effective use of external expertise; and

vi. Strengthening scientific resources.

Post-approval Monitoring Activities

The safety and efficacy of a drug submitted for approval to Health Canada is largely based on the results obtained from clinical trials conducted on the investigational drug. However, regardless of how well these trials are designed, the safety and effectiveness profile continues to evolve as the drug is used in the general population. This is referred to as the real-world drug safety and effectiveness information. Monitoring of real-world safety and effectiveness is the responsibility of Health Canada which has traditionally been restricted to assessing it with only adverse drug reaction reports. Recently the Drug Safety and effectiveness network was created within the Canadian institutes for health research (CIHR) to carry out post-approval studies.

1. Health Canada

Post-approval monitoring activities are the responsibility of the Marketed Health Products Directorate (MHPD) within Health Canada's Health Products and Food Branch (HPFB).

With respect to drugs, the Canada Vigilance Program conducts post-approval safety surveillance by collecting reports of suspected adverse drug reactions (ADRs), analyses them for risk signals and safety trends, and provides risk communications to the health care community and the public. Health professionals and consumers can submit online reports of suspected ADRs voluntarily which are then assessed by Health Canada. The program also receives ADRs from drug manufacturers, who are obligated under the Regulations to submit to Health Canada any ADR reports submitted to them. Canada Vigilance includes a publicly accessible and searchable database of all ADR reports called the Canada Vigilance Adverse Reaction Online Database.

2. The Canadian Institutes of Health Research

a. Drug safety and effectiveness network: The drug safety and effectiveness network (DSEN) within the Canadian Institutes of Health Research (CIHR), was launched in 2009, with the objective of providing evidence to support

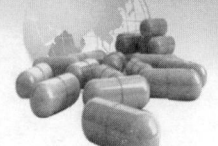

policy decisions at the federal as well as the provincial level. It is a virtual network of 150 national and international researchers which funds seven research teams in three linked collaborating center.

DSEN was created to acknowledge the limitation of pre-approval clinical trials and it provides a mechanism by which real world use of approved drugs can be analyzed. It responds to requests from drug plan managers, policy-makers, health technology assessors, and regulators to provide additional evidence on the safety and effectiveness of approved drugs.

b. Strategy for patient-oriented research: CIHR's Strategy for Patient-oriented Research (SPOR) supports a continuum of research, from initial studies in humans to comparative effectiveness and outcomes research, and the integration of this research into the health care system and clinical practice. The strategy funds researcher-initiated studies and aims to translate research findings into cost-effective health care practices with optimal outcomes.

If there is insufficient evidence to support the safety, efficacy or quality claims, the TPD will not grant a marketing authorization for the drug. All drugs granted marketing authorization in Canada are reviewed to ensure that they meet the requirements of the Food and Drugs Act.

If the TPD decides not to grant a marketing authorization, the sponsor has the opportunity to supply additional information, to re-submit its submission at a later date with additional supporting data, or to appeal the TPD's decision.

Post-approval Drug Monitoring Process

Once a new drug is on the market, regulatory controls continue. The distributor of the drug must report any new information received concerning serious side effects including failure of the drug to produce the desired effect. The distributor must also notify the TPD about any studies that have provided new safety information. The TPD monitors adverse events, investigates complaints and problem reports, maintains post-approval surveillance, and manages recalls, should the necessity arise. In addition, the TPD licenses most drug production sites and conducts regular inspections as a condition for licensing. However, certain products such as natural

S. No.	Types of submission	Days
\multicolumn{3}{c}{Table 6.2: Showing post-approval drug monitoring process}		
1.	Processing	10 Days
2.	Screening priority	25 Days
3.	Screening	45 Days
4.	NDS review—priority	180 Days
5.	NDS review—non-priority	300 Days
6.	ANDS review	180 Days

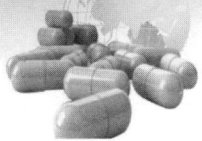

health and homeopathic remedies, some veterinary drugs and vitamin and mineral supplements are not subject to these requirements in Table 6.2.

Targeted Timelines

Drug identification numbers (DINs)—Canadian requirement

DINs are issued to all drugs approved for marketing in Canada (8 digit number generated by DPD). DIN must appear on the label.

Notices of compliance (NOC)

NOC are issued to all new drugs that are approved.

International Harmonization

HPFB has been very active in helping develop and implement international standards for the registration of new drugs. HPFB has contributed significantly to the development of over 45 harmonized technical guidelines. Canada is the only observer country to the International Conference on Harmonization (ICH) and is committed to implementing finalized ICH guidelines and standards including the common technical document (CTD).

Drug Regulatory Approval Process in the USA

In 1820, the new era of the USA drug regulation was started with the establishment of the US Pharmacopoeia. In 1906, Congress passed the original Food and Drugs Act, which require that drugs must meet official standards of strength and purity. However, in 1937, due to sulphanilamide tragedy, the Federal Food, Drug and Cosmetic Act (of 1938) was enacted and added new provisions that new drugs must be shown safe before marketing. Further, in 1962, the Kefauver-Harris Amendment Act was passed which require that manufacturers must prove that drug is safe and effective (for the claims made in labeling).

The Food and Drug Administration (FDA) is responsible for protecting and promoting public health. Like general drug approval process, FDA's new drug approval process is also accomplished in two phases: Clinical trials (CT) and new drug application (NDA) approval. FDA approval process begins only after submission of investigational new drug (IND) application. The IND application should provide high quality preclinical data to justify the testing of the drug in humans. Almost 85% of drugs are subjected to clinical trials, for which IND applications are filed. The next step is phase I clinical trials (1–3 years) on human subjects (~100). The drug's safety profile and pharmacokinetics of drug are focused in this phase. Phase II trials (2 years) are performed if the drug successfully passes phase I. To evaluate dosage, broad efficacy and additional safety in people (~300) are the main objective of the phase II. If evidence of effectiveness is shown in phase II, phase III studies (3–4 years) begins. These phase III concerns more about safety and effectiveness of drug from data of different populations, dosages and its combination with other drugs in several hundred to about 3,000 peoples.

A new drug application (NDA) can be filed only when the drug successfully

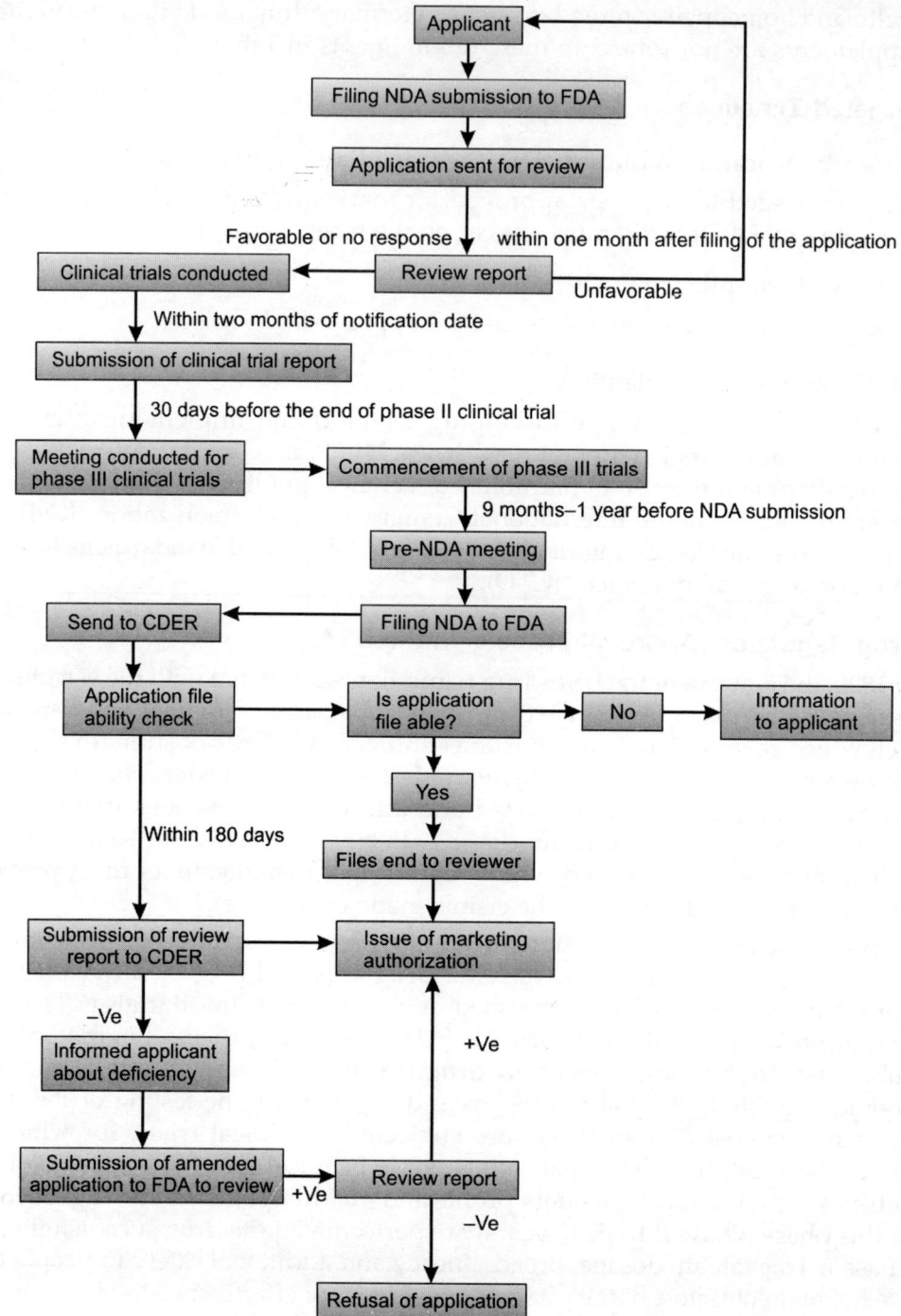

Fig. 6.9: New drug approval process of FDA in the USA

FDA—food and drug administration; NDA—new drug application; CDER—center for drug evaluation and research

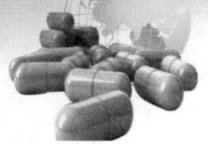

passes all three phases of clinical trials and includes all animal and human data, data analyses, pharmacokinetics of drug and its manufacturing and proposed labeling. The preclinical, clinical reports and risk-benefit analysis (product's beneficial effects outweigh its possible harmful effects) are reviewed at the center for drug evaluation and research by a team of scientists. Generally approval of an NDA is granted within two years (on an average), however, this process can be completed from two months to several years. The innovating company is allowed to market the drug after the approval of an NDA and is considered to be in phase IV trials. In this phase, new areas, uses or new populations, long-term effects, and how participants respond to different dosages are explored. Figure 6.9 represents the new drug approval process of FDA.

The prescription Drug User Fee Act of 1992 grants FDA with authorization to collect fees from users to partially cover reviewing costs of NDAs and biologics licensing applications (BLAs).

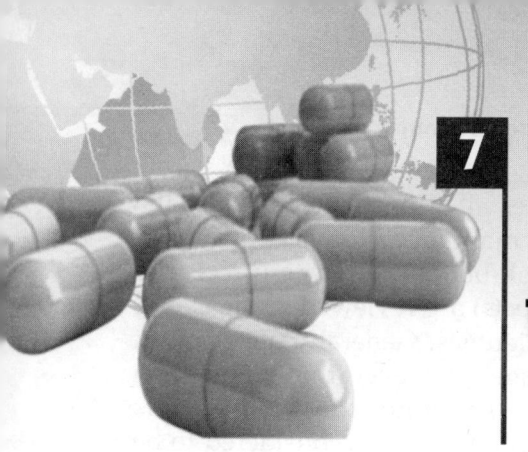

7

Drug Regulatory Approval Process for ASEAN Countries

INTRODUCTION

In our previous chapters we have studied about the drug approval process in various countries such as US, EU and Canada. The aim of the present chapter is to study the drug regulatory approval process in Association of South East Asian Nations (ASEAN) countries. A regulatory process, by which a person/organization/ sponsor/innovator gets authorization to launch a drug in the market, is known as drug approval process. Every country has its own regulatory authority, which is responsible to enforce the rules and regulations and issue the guidelines to regulate the marketing of the drugs. In the present scenario, countries have different regulatory requirements for approval of a new drug. The single regulatory approach for marketing authorization application (MAA) of a new drug product applicable to various countries (on the basis of single dossier) is utmost difficult. Therefore, the knowledge of exact and detailed regulatory requirements for MAA of each country should be known to establish a suitable regulatory strategy.

Brief Introduction to ASEAN

ASEAN was established with five founding father countries, namely Indonesia, Malaysia, Philippines, Singapore and Thailand by signing a declaration in Thailand on August 08, 1967. On Jan 08, 1984 Brunei Darussalam joined the ASEAN. On July 28, 1995 Vietnam joined the ASEAN and on July 23, 1997 Myanmar and Laos joined the ASEAN. Further on April 30, 1999 Cambodia joined the ASEAN, making up the ten member states of ASEAN. The ASEAN countries are Indonesia, Malaysia, Philippines, Singapore, Thailand, Brunei Darussalam, Vietnam, Myanmar, Laos and Cambodia (Fig. 7.1).

ACTD

ASEAN Common Technical Dossier (ACTD) is a guideline of the agreed upon common format for the preparation of a well-structured common technical dossier (CTD) applications that will be submitted to ASEAN regulatory authorities for the registration of pharmaceuticals for human use. This guideline describes a CTD format that will significantly reduce the time and resources needed to compile applications in Fig. 7.2.

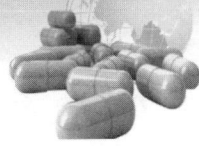

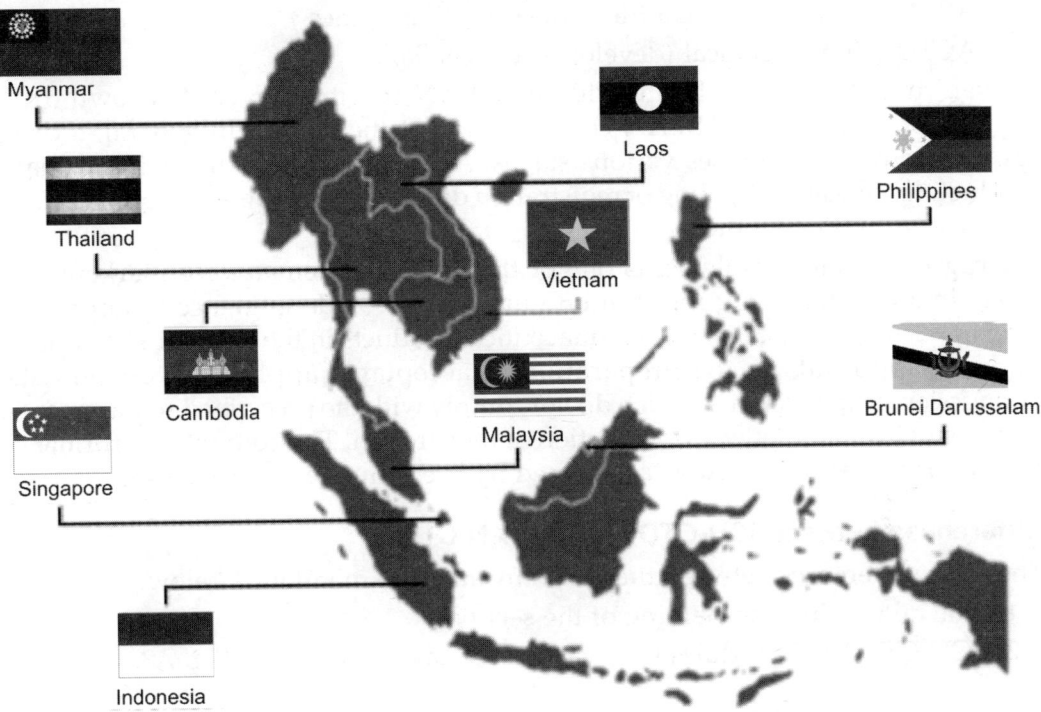

Fig. 7.1: Geographical view of 10 members ASEAN countries

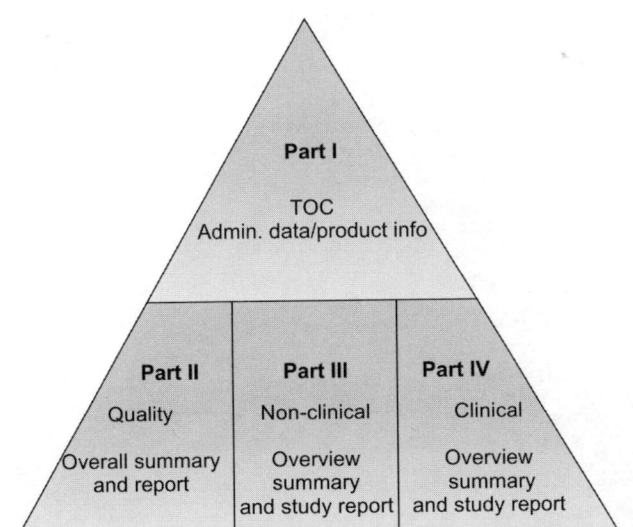

Fig. 7.2: Various parts of ASEAN common technical document

The proposed CTD is organized into four parts.

1. Overall and ACTD organization (developed by Thailand)
2. ACTD quality (developed by Indonesia)

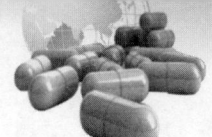

3. ACTD safety/nonclinical (developed by Philippines)
4. ACTD efficacy/clinical (developed by Thailand)

Even though some of the individual ASEAN countries have their own drug registration formats, all ASEAN countries accept the ACTD. In general, a drug approval process comprises various stages: Application to conduct clinical trials, conducting clinical trials, filing of registration dossier/new drug application (NDA) and post-marketing studies.

Drug registration implements one of the legal requirements for marketing of drugs in a country. Drug registration guidelines provide guidance to applicants who may wish to market their pharmaceutical products in the market. They intend to assist applicants in the preparation of acceptable application documents. Submission of applications, which do not comply with the prescribed requirements, may result in delays, queries or rejection of registration. **The content and format of the dossier must follow rules as defined by the competent authorities.**

Differences between ICH-CTD and ASEAN CTD

The main differences between these two formats are mentioned below:
1. The numbering and naming of the sections.
2. ICH-CTD has 5 modules whereas ACTD has 4 modules in Fig. 7.3.

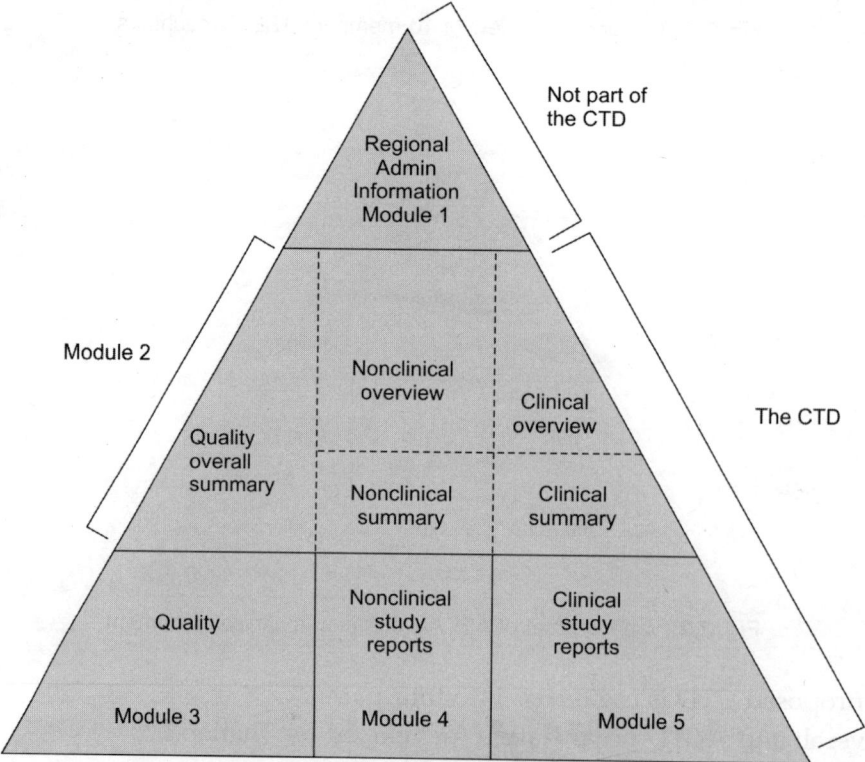

Fig. 7.3: Modules of CTD (common technical document)

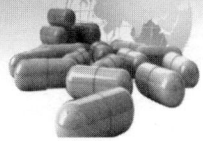

ACTD (ASEAN Common Technical Document): It is organized into four parts as follows:

1. Part I: Table of contents, administrative data and product information
2. Part II: Quality document
3. Part III: Nonclinical document
4. Part IV: Clinical document

Part I: Table of Contents, Administrative Data and Product Information

Part I contains initially the overall table of contents of the whole ACTD to provide basically the information that could be looked through respectively. Secondly, the next content is the administrative data where required specific documentation in details is put together such as application forms, label, and package insert, etc. The last section of this part is product information where necessary information includes prescribed information, mode of action, side effects, etc.

A general introduction to the pharmaceutical, including its pharmacologic class and mode of action should be included.

Section A: Introduction

Section B: Overall ASEAN common technical dossier table of contents

Section C: Documents required for registration (for example, application forms, labeling, product data sheet, prescribing information)

Part II: Quality Document

Part II should provide the overall summary followed by the study reports. The quality control document should be described in details as much as possible.

Section A: Table of contents

Section B: Quality overall summary

Section C: Body of data

1. Drug substance
2. Drug product

Part III: Nonclinical Document

Part III should provide the nonclinical overview, followed by the nonclinical written summaries and the nonclinical tabulated summaries. The document of this part is not required for generic products, minor variation products and some major variation products.

Section A: Table of contents

Section B: Nonclinical overview

Section C: Nonclinical written and tabulated summaries

1. Table of contents
2. Pharmacology
3. Pharmacokinetics
4. Toxicology

Section D: Nonclinical study reports
1. Table of contents
2. Pharmacology
3. Pharmacokinetics
4. Toxicology

Part IV: Clinical Document

Part IV should provide the clinical overview and the clinical summary. The document of this part is not required for generic products, minor variation products, and some major variation products. For ASEAN member countries, the study reports of this part may not be required for NCE, biotechnological products and other major variation products if the original products are already registered and approved for market authorization in reference countries.

Section A: Table of contents

Section B: Clinical overview

Section C: Clinical summary
1. Summary of biopharmaceutics studies and associated analytical methods
2. Summary of clinical pharmacology studies
3. Summary of clinical efficacy
4. Summary of clinical safety
5. Synopses of individual studies

Section D: Tabular listing of all clinical studies

Section E: Clinical study reports

Section F: List of key literature references

Part I: Table of Contents, Administrative Data and Product Information

Section A: Introduction

This section contains the administrative data and product information which is the Part I of the ASEAN common technical document (ACTD) for application to the drug regulatory authority.

Section B: Table of Contents
1. Application form
2. Letter of authorization (where applicable)
3. Certifications
4. Labeling
5. Product information

Section C: Guidance on the Administrative Data and Product Information
1. Application form
   English and/or official native language shall be used.

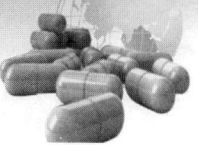

2. Letter of authorization (where applicable)
3. Certifications:
   - For contract manufacturing:
     a. License of pharmaceutical industries and contract manufacturer
     b. Contract manufacturing agreement
     c. GMP certificate of contract manufacturer
   - For manufacturing "under-license" (country specific):
     a. License of pharmaceutical industries
     b. GMP certificate of the manufacturer
     c. Copy of "under-license" agreement.
   - For locally manufactured products (excluding the above):
     a. License of pharmaceutical industries
     b. GMP certificate (country specific)
   - For imported products:
     a. License of pharmaceutical industries/importer/wholesaler (country specific)
     b. Certificate of pharmaceutical product issued by the competent authority in the country of origin according to the current WHO format
     c. Site master file of manufacturer (unless previously submitted within the last 2 years) (country specific)
4. Labeling
   English and/or official native language shall be used.
5. Product information
   5.1. Package insert
        English and/or official native language shall be used.
        Package insert is required for generic products
   5.2. Summary of product characteristics (product data sheet)
        English and/or official native language shall be used.
        Summary of product characteristics is required for NCE and biotechnology products.
   5.3. Patient information leaflet (PIL)
        English and/or official native language shall be used.
        PIL is required for over-the-counter products

Part II. Quality Document

Section A: Table of Contents
A table of contents for the filled application should be provided.

Section B: Quality Overall Summary
Table 7.1 Gives a view of the quality overall summary of Part II of ACTD.

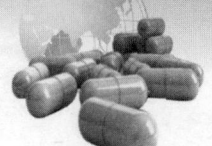

Table 7.1: Quality overall summary of Part II of ACTD	
S drug substance	*P drug product*
S1 General information	P1 Description and composition
S2 Manufacture	P2 Pharmaceutical development
S3 Characterization	P3 Manufacture
S4 Control of drug substance	P4 Control of excipients
S5 Reference standards or materials	P5 Control of finished product
S6 Container closure	P6 Reference standards or materials
S7 Stability	P7 Container closure
	P8 Stability
	P9 Product interchangeability equivalence evidence

Section C: Body of data

S1 General information
S1.1 Nomenclature
S1.2 Structural formula
S1.3 General properties

S2 Manufacture
S2.1 Manufacture(s)
S2.2 Description of manufacturing process and process controls
S2.3 Control of materials
S2.4 Control of critical steps and intermediates
S2.5 Process validation and/or evaluation
S2.6 Manufacturing process development

S3 Characterization
S3.1 Elucidation of structure and characteristic
S3.2 Impurities

S4 Control of drug substance
S4.1 Specification
S4.2 Analytical procedures
S4.3 Validation of analytical procedures
S4.4 Batch analysis
S4.5 Justification of specification

S5 Reference standards or materials

S6 Container closure system

S7 Stability

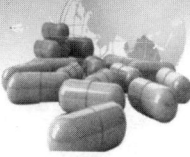

P Drug Product

P1 Description and composition

P2 Pharmaceutical development

P2.1 Information on development studies

P2.2 Component of drug product

P2.3 Finished product

P2.4 Manufacturing process development

P2.5 Container closure system

P2.6 Microbiological attributes

P2.7 Compatibility

P3 Manufacture

P3.1 Batch formula

P3.2 Manufacturing process and process control

P3.3 Controls of critical steps and intermediates

P3.4 Process validation and/or evaluation

P4 Control of excipients

P4.1 Specification

P4.2 Analytical procedures

P4.3 Excipients of human and animal origin

P4.4 Novel excipients

P5 Control of finished product

P5.1 Specification

P5.2 Analytical procedures

P5.3 Validation of analytical procedures

P5.4 Batch analyses

P5.5 Characterization of impurities

P5.6 Justification of specification

P6 Reference standards or materials

P7 Container closure system

P8 Product stability

P9 Product interchangeability

PART III: Nonclinical Document

Section A. Table of Contents

Guide on nonclinical overviews and summaries

This guide provides recommendations for the harmonization of the nonclinical overview, nonclinical written and tabulated summaries.

The primary purpose of nonclinical written and tabulated summaries should be to provide a comprehensive, factual synopsis of the nonclinical data. The interpretation of the data, the clinical relevance of the findings, cross-linking with the quality aspects of the pharmaceutical, and the implications of the nonclinical findings for the safe use of the pharmaceutical (i.e. as applicable to labeling) should be addressed in the nonclinical overview.

Section B: Nonclinical Overview

The nonclinical overview should provide an integrated, overall analysis of the information in the common technical document.

1. *General aspects*

The nonclinical overview should present an integrated and critical assessment of the pharmacologic, pharmacokinetic, and toxicological evaluation of the pharmaceutical. Where relevant guidance on the conduct of studies exists, these should be taken into consideration, and any deviation from these guidance should be discussed and justified. The nonclinical testing strategy should be discussed and justified. There should comment on the good laboratory practice (GLP) status of the studies submitted. Any association between nonclinical findings and the quality characteristics of the human pharmaceutical, the results of clinical trials, or effects seen with related products should be indicated, as appropriate.

Except for biotechnology-derived products, an assessment of the impurities and degradants present in the drug substance and product should be included, along with what is known of their potential pharmacologic and toxicological effects. This assessment should form part of the justification for proposed impurity limits in the drug substance and product and be appropriately cross-referenced to the quality documentation. The implications of any differences in the chirality, chemical form, and impurity profile between the compound used in the nonclinical studies and the product to be marketed should be discussed. For biotechnology-derived products, comparability of material used in nonclinical and clinical studies and proposed for marketing should be assessed. If a drug product includes a novel excipient, an assessment of the information regarding the excipient's safety should be provided.

Relevant, scientific literature and the properties of related products should be taken into account. If details references to published, scientific literature are to be used in place of studies conducted by the applicant, this should be supported by an appropriate justification that reviews the design of the studies and any deviations from available guidance. In addition, the availability of information on the quality of batches of drug substances used in these referenced studies should be discussed.

2. *Content and structural format*

The nonclinical overview should be presented in the following sequence:

Nonclinical overview

1. Overview of the nonclinical testing strategy
2. Pharmacology
3. Pharmacokinetics

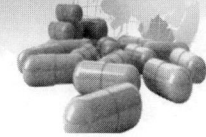

4. Toxicology

5. Integrated overview and conclusion

6. List of literature citations

Studies conducted to establish the pharmacodynamic effects, the mode of action, and potential side effects should be evaluated, and consideration should be given to the significance of any issues that arise.

The assessment of the pharmacokinetic, toxic kinetic, and metabolism data should address the relevance of the analytical methods used, the pharmacokinetic models, and the derived parameters. It might be appropriate to cross-refer to more detailed consideration of certain issues within the pharmacology or toxicology studies (e.g. impact of the disease states, changes in physiology, ant product antibodies, cross-pieces consideration of toxic kinetic data). Inconsistencies in the data should be discussed. Inter-species comparisons of metabolism and systemic exposure comparisons in animals and humans (AUC, Cmax, and other appropriate parameters) should be discussed and the limitations and utility of the nonclinical studies for prediction of potential adverse effects in humans highlighted.

Section C: Nonclinical Written and Tabulated Summaries

1. *Guidance on nonclinical written summaries*

   1.1. Introduction

   This guidance is intended to assist authors in the preparation of nonclinical pharmacology, pharmacokinetics and toxicology written summaries in an appropriate format. This guidance is not intended to indicate what studies required. It merely indicates an appropriate format for the nonclinical data that have been acquired.

   1.2. General presentation issues

   Order of presentation of information within sections

   When available, *in vitro* studies should precede *in vivo* studies. Where multiple studies of the same type are summarized within the pharma-cokinetics and toxicology sections, studies should be ordered by species, by route, and then by duration (shortest duration first).

2. *Content of nonclinical written and tabulated summaries*

   The aim of this section should be to introduce the reviewer to the pharmaceutical and to its proposed clinical use. The following key elements should be covered:

   i. Brief information concerning the pharmaceutical's structure (preferably, a structure diagram should be provided) and pharmacologic properties.

   ii. Information concerning the pharmaceutical's proposed clinical indication, dose, and duration of use.

   2.1. Pharmacology

   a. Written summary

   b. Within the pharmacology written summary, the data should be presented in the following sequence:

   i. Brief summary
   ii. Primary pharmacodynamics
   iii. Secondary pharmacodynamics
   iv. Safety pharmacology
   v. Pharmacodynamic drug interactions
   vi. Discussion and conclusion
   vii. Tables and figures (either here or included in text)
 2.2. Pharmacokinetics
  a. Written summary
  b. The sequence of the pharmacokinetics written summary should be as follows:
   i. Brief summary
   ii. Method of analysis
   iii. Absorption
   iv. Distribution
   v. Metabolism
   vi. Excretion
   vii. Pharmacokinetic drug interactions
   viii. Other pharmacokinetic studies
   ix. Discussion and conclusion
   x. Tables and figures (either here or included in text)
 2.3 Toxicology
  a. Written summary
  b. The sequence of the toxicology written summary should be as follows:
   i. Brief summary
   ii. Single-dose toxicity
   iii. Repeat-dose toxicity
   iv. Genotoxicity
   v. Carcinogenicity
   vi. Reproductive and developmental toxicity
   vii. Studies in juvenile animals
   viii. Local tolerance
   ix. Other toxicity studies
   x. Discussion and conclusions
   xi. Tables and figures (either here or included in text)

3. *Guidance on nonclinical tabulated summaries*

It is recommended that summary tables for the nonclinical information in the common technical document be provided in the format outlined in this guidance. Applicants can modify the format, if warranted, to provide the best possible presentation of the information and to facilitate the understanding and evaluation of the results.

This guidance is not intended to indicate what studies are requested, but solely to advise how to tabulate study results if a study is performed. Applicants can add some items to or delete some items from the cited format, where

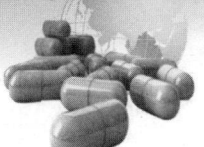

appropriate. One tabular format can contain results from several studies. Alternatively, it may be appropriate to cite the data resulting from one study in several tabular formats.

Section D: Nonclinical Study Reports

For ASEAN member countries, the study reports of this part may not be required for NCE, biotechnological products and other major variation products if the original products are already registered and approved for market authorization in reference countries. This guidance presents an agreed upon format for the organization of the nonclinical reports in the common technical document for applications that will be submitted to regulatory authorities. This guidance is not intended to indicate what studies are required. It merely indicates an appropriate format for the nonclinical data that have been acquired.

1. Table of contents

   A table of contents should be provided that lists all of the nonclinical study reports and gives the location of each study report in the common technical document.

2. Pharmacology

   2.1. Written study reports

   The study reports should be presented in the following order:
   i. Primary pharmacodynamics
   ii. Secondary pharmacodynamics
   iii. Safety pharmacology
   iv. Pharmacodynamic drug interactions

3. Pharmacokinetics

   3.1. Written study reports

   The study reports should be presented in the following order:
   i. Analytical methods and validation reports (if separate reports are available)
   ii. Absorption
   iii. Distribution
   iv. Metabolism
   v. Excretion
   vi. Pharmacokinetic drug interactions (nonclinical)
   vii. Other pharmacokinetic studies

4. Toxicology

   4.1. Written study reports

   The study reports should be presented in the following order:
   a. Single-dose toxicity (in order by species, by route)
   b. Repeat-dose toxicity (in order by species, by route, by duration, including supportive toxic kinetics evaluations)
   c. Genotoxicity
      i. *In vitro*
      ii. *In vivo* (including supportive toxic kinetics evaluations)

    d. Carcinogenicity (including supportive toxic kinetics evaluations):

        i. Long-term studies (in order by species, including range-finding studies that cannot appropriately be included under repeat-dose toxicity or pharmacokinetics)

       ii. Short- or medium-term studies (including range-finding studies that cannot appropriately be included under repeat-dose toxicity or pharmacokinetics)

     iii. Other studies

    e. Reproductive and developmental toxicity (including range-finding studies and supportive toxic kinetics evaluations) (If modified study designs are used, the following subheadings should be modified accordingly):

        i. Fertility and early embryonic development

       ii. Embryo fetal development

     iii. Prenatal and postnatal development, including maternal function

     iv. Studies in which offspring (juvenile animals) are dosed and/or further evaluated

    f. Local tolerance

    g. Other toxicity studies (if available):

        i. Antigenicity

       ii. Immunotoxicity

     iii. Mechanistic studies (if not included elsewhere)

     iv. Dependence

      v. Metabolites

     vi. Impurities

    vii. Other

Part IV: Clinical Document

Section A: Table of Contents

A table of contents for the filled application should be provided.

Section B: Clinical Overview

The clinical overview is intended to provide a critical analysis of the clinical data in the ASEAN Common Technical Dossier (ACTD). The clinical overview is primarily intended for use by regulatory agencies in the review of the clinical section of a marketing application. It should also be a useful reference to the overall clinical findings for regulatory agency staff involved in the review of other sections of the marketing application. The clinical overview should present the strengths and limitations of the development program and study results, analyze the benefits and risks of the medicinal product in the intended use, and describe how the study results support clinical parts of the prescribing information.

In order to achieve these objectives the clinical overview should:

    i. Describe and explain the overall approach to the clinical development of a medicinal product, including critical study design decisions.

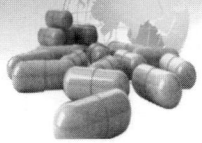

ii. Assess the quality of the design and performance of the studies, and include a statement regarding GCP compliance.

iii. Provide a brief overview of the clinical findings, including important limitations.

iv. Provide an evaluation of benefits and risks based upon the conclusion of the relevant clinical studies, including interpretation of how the efficacy and safety findings support the proposed dose and target indication and an evaluation of how prescribing information and other approaches will optimize benefits and manage risks.

v. Address particular efficacy or safety issues encountered in development, and how they have been evaluated and resolved.

vi. Explore unresolved issues, explain why they should not be considered as barriers to approval, and describe plans to resolve them.

vii. Explain the basis for important or unusual aspects of the prescribing information.

Table of contents for the clinical overview:

i. Product development rationale

ii. Overview of biopharmaceutics

iii. Overview of clinical pharmacology

iv. Overview of efficacy

v. Overview of safety

vi. Benefits and risks conclusion

Section C: Clinical Summary

For ASEAN member countries, the clinical study reports of this part may not be required for NCE, biotechnological products and other major variation products if the original products are already registered and approved for market authorization in reference countries. Therefore, the authority who wishes to obtain such clinical study reports should request for additional documentation.

The clinical summary is intended to provide a detailed, factual summarization of all the clinical information in the ASEAN common technical dossier. This includes information provided in clinical study reports; information obtained from any meta-analyses or other cross study analyses for which full reports have been included in clinical study reports and post-marketing data for products that have been marketed in other regions. The comparisons and analyses of results across studies provided in this document should focus on factual observations.

Table of contents for the clinical summary:

i. Summary of biopharmaceutical studies and associated analytical methods

ii. Summary of clinical pharmacology studies

iii. Summary of clinical efficacy

iv. Summary of clinical safety

v. Synopsis of individual studies

Section D: Tabular Listing of All Clinical Studies

Section E: Clinical Study Reports

For ASEAN member countries, the clinical study reports of this part may not be required for NCE, biotechnological products and other major variation products if the original products are already registered and approved for market authorization in reference countries. Therefore, the authority who requires specific study reports should ask for the necessary documents. The ICH E3 provides guidance on the organization of clinical study reports, other clinical data, and references within the ASEAN Common Technical Dossier (ACTD) for registration of a pharmaceutical product for human use.

Section F: List of Key Literature References

List of referenced documents, including important published articles, official meeting minutes, or other regulatory guidance or advice should be provided here.

Drug Registration and Approval Process in Singapore:

The major Drug Laws governing in Singapore are mentioned below:

1. Medicines Act
2. Poisons Act
3. Misuse of Drugs Act
4. Sale of Drugs Act
5. Medicines (Advertisement and Sale) Act

As per Medicines Act, licensing authority (Chief Executive of the **Health Sciences Authority (HSA)** have the authority to grant, renew, vary, suspend and revoke licenses and certificates.

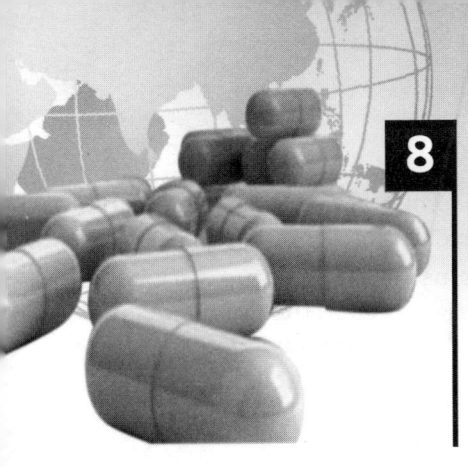

8

Drug Regulatory Approval Process for Emerging Economies

Emerging economies are important and expanding globally and they play important role for general and lifesaving drugs. Emerging economies consists of mainly the countries from Asia Pacific, Latin America, Eastern Europe, Africa and Gulf countries. These countries are not differing in their region but also in many other aspects as regulation of pharmaceuticals, using different guidelines for registration, registration fees, requirements to maintain registration, patent regulation and legislation for the drug.

From the perspective of the biopharmaceutical industry, the definition of emerging markets also continues to evolve. Most major companies have either created or reorganized their groups to focus on emerging markets based on the market size or market potential rather than by regulatory systems. However, from a regulatory perspective, the definition and demarcation of "emerging markets" is rather straightforward. Generally, from the regulatory affairs perspective, the world is broken down into "primary markets" and "secondary markets". The primary markets are those where the regulatory agencies conduct complete evaluation of safety, efficacy and quality of the product (usually the original ICH countries). The secondary markets are the countries which depend on the approval of the "primary countries" and generally require a Certificate of Pharmaceutical Product (CPP).

From the content perspective, the primary countries would get the full content as per the ICH guidelines. For the "secondary countries", which are also referred to as the "emerging countries" or "rest of the world", the dossier would be a stripped-down version of the full common technical document (CTD).

DRUG REGULATORY APPROVAL PROCESS FOR EMERGING ECONOMIES

Drug Regulatory Approval Process in India

Introduction

Current federal law requires that a drug be the subject of an approved marketing application before it is transported or distributed across state lines. Because a sponsor will probably want to ship the investigational drug to clinical investigators in many

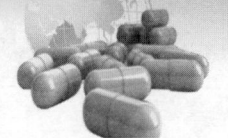

states, it must seek an exemption from that legal requirement. The IND is the means through which the sponsor technically obtains this exemption from the FDA.

FDA's role in the development of a new drug begins when the drug's sponsor (usually the manufacturer or potential marketer) having screened the new molecule for pharmacological activity and acute toxicity potential in animals, wants to test its diagnostic or therapeutic potential in humans. At that point, the molecule changes in legal status under the Federal Food, Drug, and Cosmetic Act and becomes a new drug subject to specific requirements of the drug regulatory system.

The IND application must contain information in three broad areas:

1. *Animal pharmacology and toxicology studies*: Preclinical data to permit an assessment as to whether the product is reasonably safe for initial testing in humans. Also included are any previous experience with the drug in humans (often foreign use).

2. *Manufacturing information*: Information pertaining to the composition, manufacturer, stability, and controls used for manufacturing the drug substance and the drug product. This information is assessed to ensure that the company can adequately produce and supply consistent batches of the drug.

3. *Clinical protocols and investigator information*: Detailed protocols for proposed clinical studies to assess whether the initial-phase trials will expose subjects to unnecessary risks. Also, information on the qualifications of clinical investigators-professionals (generally physicians) who oversee the administration of the experimental compound to assess whether they are qualified to fulfill their clinical trial duties. Finally, commitments to obtain informed consent from the research subjects, to obtain review of the study by an institutional review board (IRB), and to adhere to the investigational new drug regulations.

Once the IND is submitted, the sponsor must wait 30 calendar days before initiating any clinical trials. During this time, FDA has an opportunity to review the IND for safety to assure that research subjects will not be subjected to unreasonable risk.

Overview of Drug Regulatory Approval Process

The India's parliament passed the Drug and Cosmetic Act 1940 and Rules 1945 for the regulation of import, manufacture, distribution and sale of drugs and cosmetics. The Central Drugs Standard Control Organization (CDSCO), and the office of its leader, the Drugs Controller General (India) [DCGI] was established.

The Indian government added schedule Y to the Drug and Cosmetic Rules 1945 in 1988 which provides the guidelines and requirements for clinical trials, which was further revised in 2005 to bring it at same level with globally established procedure. The changes includes, establishing definitions for Phase I–IV trials and clear responsibilities for investigators and sponsors.

In 2006 the clinical trials were further divided into two groups. In one group (category A) clinical trials are conducted and other markets with capable and adult regulatory systems whereas the remaining are fall into another group (category B) other than A.

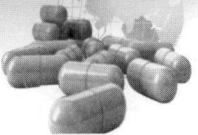

Clinical trials of category A (approved in the US, Britain, Switzerland, Australia, Canada, Germany, South Africa, Japan and the European Union) are appropriate for fast tracking in India, and are expected to be accepted within 2 months. The clinical trials of category B are under more analysis and approve within 16 to 18 weeks.

An application for the conduction of clinical trials in India should be submitted along with the data of chemistry, manufacturing, control and animal studies to DCGI. The date of the trial protocol, investigator's brochures, and informed consent documents should also be attached with the application. One copy of the application must be submitted to the ethical committee and after the approval of DCGI and ethical committee the clinical trials are conducted to determine the maximum tolerated dose in humans, adverse reactions, etc.

The Phase I clinical trials are conducted on healthy human volunteers. The therapeutic uses and effective dose ranges are determined in Phase II trials in 10–12 patients at each dose level. The Phase III trials (confirmatory trials) are conducted to generate data regarding the efficacy and safety of the drug in ~ 100 patients (at 3–4 centers) to verify efficacy and safety claims and Phase III trials should be conducted on a minimum of 500 patients spread across 10–15 centers, if the new drug substance is not marketed in any other country.

After the completion of clinical trials the new drug registration (using form # 44 along with full preclinical and clinical testing information) is applied. The full information on the market condition of the drug in other countries is also required other than the information on safety and efficacy. The information regarding the prescription, samples and testing protocols, product monograph, labels, and cartons must also be submitted.

The application can be review in 12–18 months. Figure 8.1 shows the new drug approval process of India. After approved by the NDA, when a company is permitted to distribute and market the product, it is considered to be in Phase IV trials, in which new uses or new populations, long-term effects, etc. are explored.

The drug approval process differentiates from one country to another. In some countries, only a single body regulates the drugs and is responsible for all regulatory job such as approval of new drugs, issuing license for manufacturing and inspection of manufacturing plants, e.g. in the USA, FDA performs all the functions. While in some counties all jobs are not performed by a single regulatory authority, such as in India, this responsibility is divided on Centralized and State authorities. The other issues where the difference appears are, time taken for the sanction of a CTA application, time taken in appraisal of marketing authorization application, registration fee, registration process and marketing exclusivity.

Some counties have two different appraisal processes as normal review process and accelerated review process as in the USA, China, etc. and some countries have only a single appraisal process as in India. Similarly, the design used for the presentation of file submitted for approval of drug is also different.

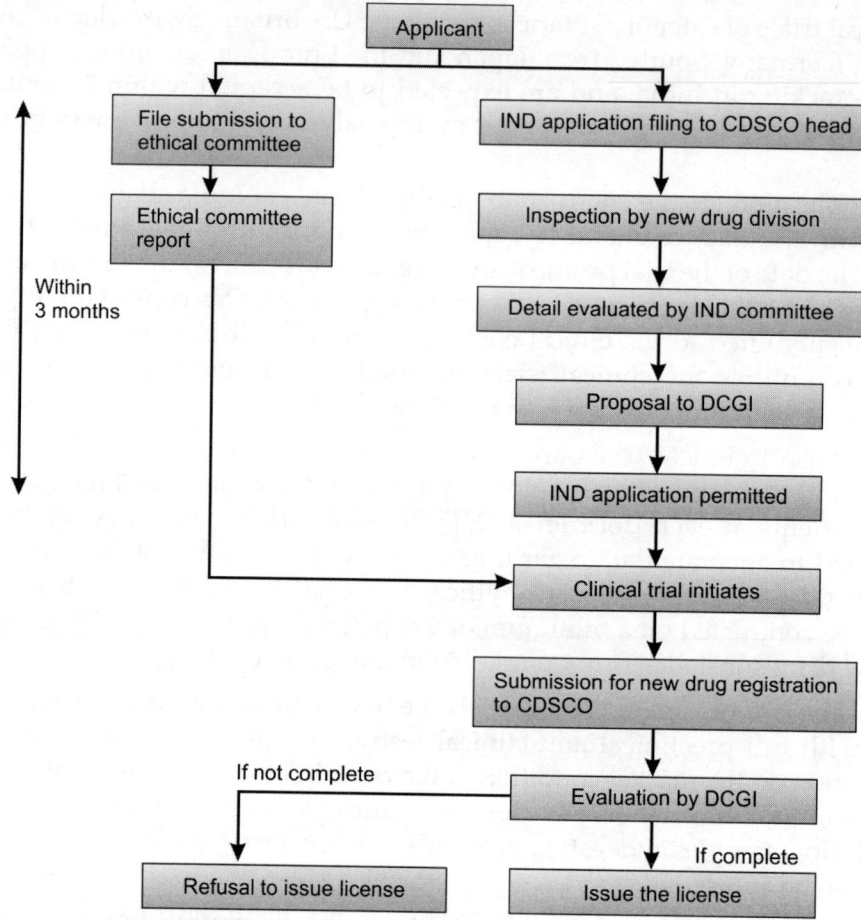

Fig. 8.1: New drug registration process of India

IND—investigational new drug; DCGI—Drug Controller General of India; CDSCO—Central Drug Standards Control Organization

CTD Guideline in INDIA

This guideline applies to import/manufacture and marketing approval of new drugs including new chemical entity, new indication, new dosage forms, modified release form, new route of administration, etc. under the definition of new drug under Rule 122E of Drugs and Cosmetics rules as a finished pharmaceutical product.

The CTD is only a format for submission of information to CDSCO. It does not define the content. CDSCO also adopted the CTD.

Module 1: General Information

This module should contain documents specific to India; for example, Form 44, Treasury challan fee or the proposed label for use in India.

1. Covering letters and comprehensive table of contents (module 1 to 5)

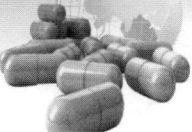

2. Administrative information
   - Brief introduction about the applicant company
   - Duly filled and signed application form 44 and treasury challan
   - Legal and critical documents
   - Coordinates related to the application
   - General information of the drug product
   - Summary of the testing protocol(s) for quality control testing
   - Regulatory status in other countries
   - Domestic price of the drug followed in the countries of origin
   - Brief profile of manufacturer's company and business activity
   - Information regarding involvement of expert if any
   - Samples of drug product
   - Promotional material

Module 2: CTD Summaries

This module should begin with a general introduction to the pharmaceutical, including its pharmacologic class, mode of action, and proposed clinical use, not exceeding one page. Module 2 should contain 7 sections in the following order:

1. CTD table of contents
2. CTD introduction
3. Quality overall summary
4. Nonclinical overview
5. Clinical overview
6. Nonclinical written and tabulated summaries
7. Clinical summary

In this module following information is required:

1. Table of content of module
2. Introduction
3. Quality overall summary
4. Summary of drug substance and drug product
5. Nonclinical overview
6. Clinical overview

Module 3: Quality

In this module following information is required:

1. Table of contents of module 3
2. Drug substances
3. Manufacture of drug substances
4. Characterization of drug substances
5. Quality control of drug substances
6. Reference standards and material
7. Container closer system

8. Stability of drug substance
9. Drug product and manufacture of drug product
10. Control of drugs product and excipient

Module 4: Nonclinical Study Report

Table of contents in this module should be provided that lists all of the nonclinical study reports and gives the location of the each study reports in CTD.
It contains following data:

1. Study reports
   - Pharmacology
   - Toxicology
2. Literature references

Module 5: Clinical Study Report

It contains tabular listing of all clinical studies. Following data are required:

1. Clinical study report
2. Reports of biopharmaceutical studies
3. Reports of studies pertinent to pharmacokinetic using human biomaterials
4. Reports of human pharmacokinetic studies
5. Reports of human pharmacodynamic studies
6. Reports of efficacy and safety study
7. Reports of post-marketing experience
8. Case report form and individual patient listing
9. Literature references (CDSCO guideline)

Drug Regulatory Approval Process in China

The Chinese Ministry of Health planned drug regulation in 1963, for the management of new drugs. The China's State Pharmaceutical Administration in association with Ministry of Health in 1979, published the New Drug Management Regulations. The first comprehensive Drug Administrative Law was framed in 1985 in vision of protecting the public health and promoting the economic developments in pharmaceuticals. This law was amended in 1999 by two additional provisions for new drug approval and provisions for new biological product approval. The sanction process of new drug applications (NDA) includes enough preclinical data for verification of drug's safety and validation of the initiation of clinical trials. In 2001 the Drug Administrative Law was further revised requiring premarket testing, sanction for new drug products, and prohibits drug adulteration.

The State Food and Drug Administration (SFDA) is authorized by the drug administrative law to approve new drugs for marketing. The new drug registration process also contains the clinical study application and the new drug applications. The provincial drug administration authorities (PDAAs) should arrange the works of the official review of submitted materials, i.e. on-site examination and sampling

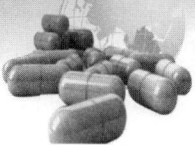

just after receiving the drug registration application. The aim behind this official review is to assure the content and format of the submitted materials is in line with the requirements and all the required materials have been submitted. After this review, the PDAAs send the qualified applications to the SFDA for further review and the import drug registration application should be straight submitted to SFDA by the applicant. SFDA's Department of Drug Registration carefully reviews the totality of the submitted materials, files the qualified applications and transmits all the materials of qualified applications to the center for drug evaluation (CDE) directly attracted to SFDA. The CDE decide whether the safety and effectiveness information submitted for a new drug are sufficient for manufacturing and marketing approval and send the review report to SFDA. SFDA carefully consider the recommendations and review the results of CDE and decides whether the drug registration is done or not. The application can be approved and issues the certificate of drug approval and drug approval number to the qualified applicant. Figures 8.2 and 8.3 show the new drug approval process and clinical trial approval process of China, respectively.

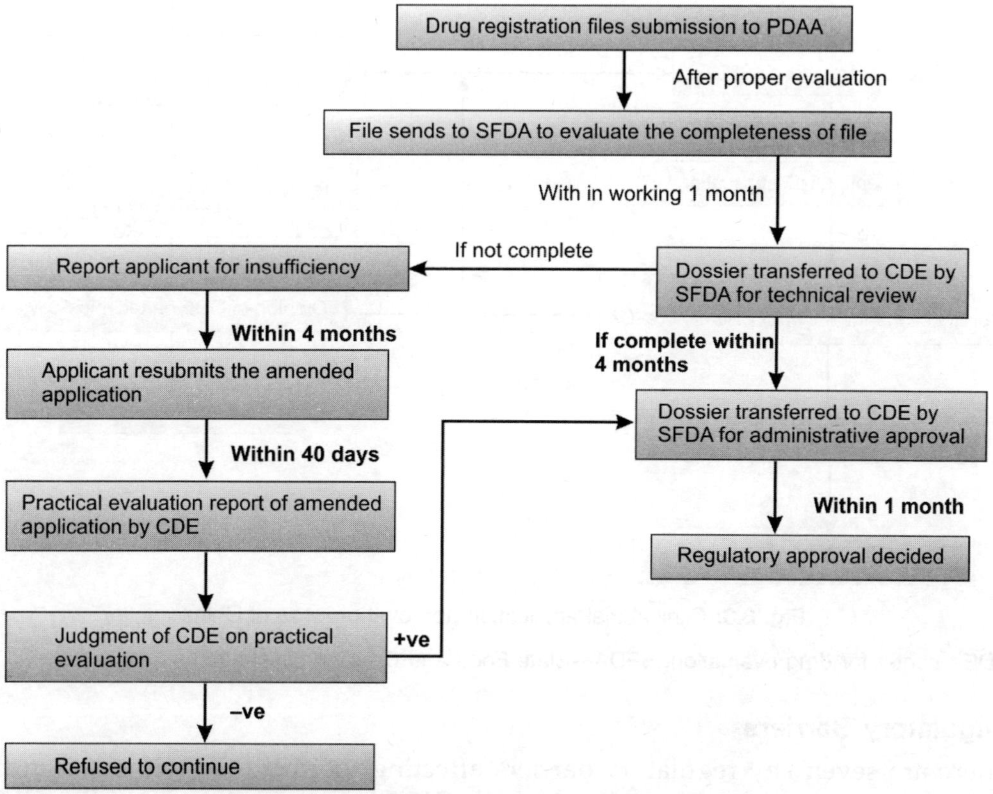

Drug registration files submission to PDAA

After proper evaluation

File sends to SFDA to evaluate the completeness of file

With in working 1 month

If not complete

Report applicant for insufficiency

Dossier transferred to CDE by SFDA for technical review

Within 4 months

If complete within 4 months

Applicant resubmits the amended application

Dossier transferred to CDE by SFDA for administrative approval

Within 40 days

Within 1 month

Practical evaluation report of amended application by CDE

Regulatory approval decided

Judgment of CDE on practical evaluation   +ve

−ve

Refused to continue

Fig. 8.2: New drug registration process of China

PDAA—provincial drug administration authority

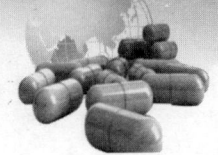

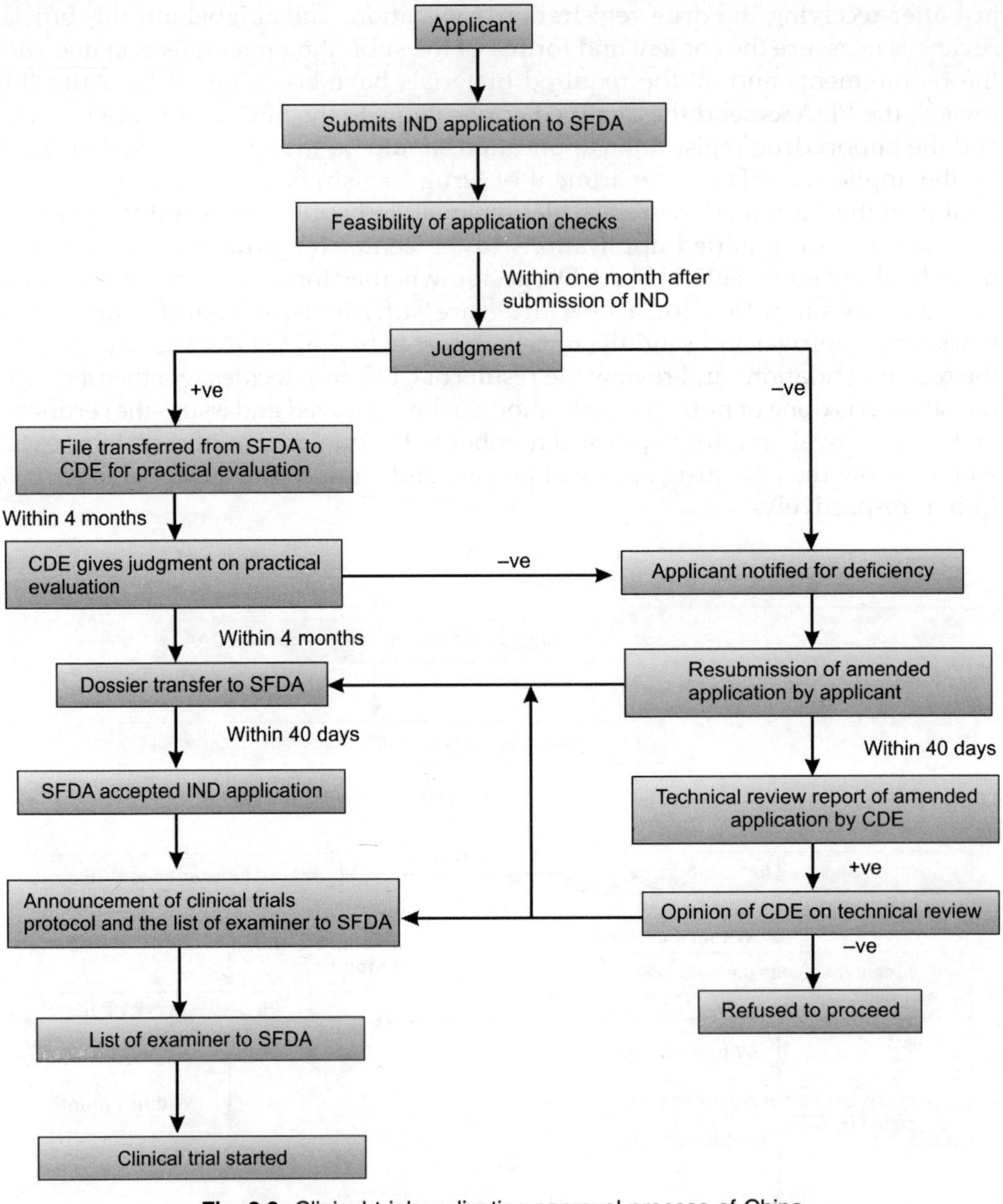

```
                        ┌─────────────────┐
                        │    Applicant    │
                        └────────┬────────┘
                                 ▼
                 ┌───────────────────────────────┐
                 │  Submits IND application to SFDA │
                 └───────────────┬───────────────┘
                                 ▼
                 ┌───────────────────────────────┐
                 │ Feasibility of application checks │
                 └───────────────┬───────────────┘
                                 │    Within one month after
                                 │    submission of IND
                                 ▼
                        ┌─────────────────┐
                        │    Judgment     │
                        └─────────────────┘
```

Fig. 8.3: Clinical trial application approval process of China

CDE—center for drug evaluation, SFDA—State Food and Drug Administration

Regulatory Barriers

There are seven key regulatory barriers affecting the drug lag witnessed in the developing economies. These barriers are Western approval, LCD, CPP, GMP, pricing approval, document authentication and harmonization. These barriers need to be overcome in order to reduce drug lag further in the future.

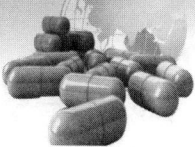

1. Western approval

There have been a few instances to date where a drug has been granted its first worldwide approval in a developing economy. This could be due to the additional testing requirements that these countries have in order to comply with their local guidelines. In order to submit an MAA in the developing economies, companies usually have to wait for an established regulatory authority such as the FDA or EMA to grant approval of that drug. The reliance on these western countries has led to this barrier being labeled as 'Western approval'.

2. LCD

LCD is currently required by China and India at Phase III. The emerging markets have sometimes not been highly regarded enough to be included in global clinical development (GCD) due to lack of infrastructure and resources. Different ethnicities have different metabolisms which can sometimes mean variations in the actions of drugs on patients. Some of the most developed economic countries such as China, India and Korea have thus decided that they need LCD in order to protect their populations. To carry out LCD, an investigational new drug (IND) application has to be approved as a consequence of positive results, a new drug application (NDA) is submitted in that country and a full MAA review can then be undertaken. LCD was formerly carried out sequentially to GCD, which led to very extreme drug lags. It is preferable for it to be in parallel with, or part of, GCD which has helped to reduce the lag to some extent. GCD has expanded widely in recent years and so LCD may become irrelevant and costly in terms of extra resources.

3. CPP

The World Health Organization (WHO) primarily devised CPPs as a way of enabling regulatory authorities to ascertain the GMP and quality status of the drug product which has been submitted for MAA review. It helps to establish that the drug product in the approval market is the same quality as that of the product which is being imported. A CPP also provides information on the product itself and its regulatory status in the issuing market. A CPP can be issued by an authority when a drug receives approval in that country and may be required for product submission or approval in another country. However, the FDA will not issue a CPP unless the product will be exported from within the US. For authorities requiring a CPP at the time of submission, the applicant company has to wait for the issuing country to have approved the drug which can take up to 18 months, thus significantly delaying registration in the new market. The time taken to issue a CPP varies between authorities but may take from 2 weeks up to 9 months.

4. GMP

Most WHO CPPs carry a GMP statement but some recipient authorities continue to request a separate GMP certificate which is an unnecessary duplication and waste of resources.

5. Pricing approval

Price certificate requirement is another important barrier. Price certificates are an agreement between the pharmaceutical company and health authority as to the price at which the drug will be sold when MA is granted. The review and approval process for pricing is sometimes integrated into that of the MAA review, delaying the latter further. In order to reduce drug lag, it would be preferable to carry out these processes separately, particularly as they have different focuses—the drug review process being scientific and the pricing review process being policy based. It is thus the pricing approval and negotiation that is the source of the time delay with the price certificate just being a tool used within that process.

6. Document authentication

Authorities can request that CPPs, GMP and price certificates are legalized and notarized. Notarization can take only a few weeks to be carried out—this is done by a notary, of which most companies now have their own. Legalization, however, is a lengthy process. It is granted by the embassy of the importing country based in the exporting country and can take many months, but it is dependent on the legislation of the exporting country.

7. Harmonization

It is evident that a lack of harmonization between countries can lead to 'unnecessary duplication of effort' and a 'waste of valuable resources'. In short, this can increase drug lag.

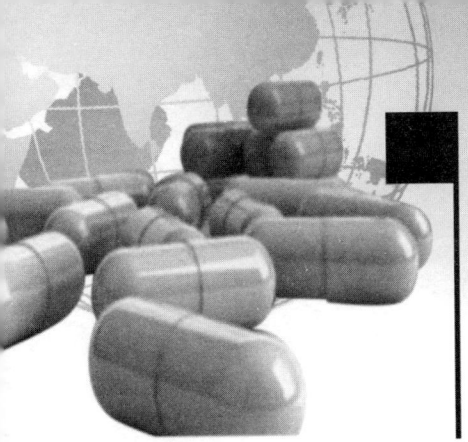

Glossary

AADA: Abbreviated antibiotic drug application

AAP: Accelerated assessment procedure

AAPS: American Association of Pharmaceutical Scientists

ABHI: Association of British Healthcare Industries (medical devices sector)

ACRP: Association of Clinical Research Professionals

ACTD: ASEAN common technical dossier (*see* **ASEAN**)

ACVM: Agricultural compounds and veterinary medicines (New Zealand)

ADC: Additional data collection

ADE: Adverse device event (AE judged to be related to the medical device)

ADEC: Australian Drug Evaluation Committee

AEMPS: Agencia Española de Medicamentos y Productos Sanitarios (Spain)

AEPAR: Associación Española de Profesionales de Actividades de Registro (Spanish Regulatory Affairs Association)

AERS: Adverse event reporting system (US FDA)

AESGP: Association Européenne des Spécialitiés Pharmaceutiques Grand Public (Association of the European Self-Medication Industry)

AFAR: Association Française des Affaires Reglémentaires (French Regulatory Affairs Association)

AFDO: Association of Food and Drug Officials (US)

AFMPS: Agence Fédérale des Médicaments et des Produits de Santé (Belgium)

AHSC: Academic health science centre (UK)

AI: Adverse incident (medical devices sector)

AIFA: Agenzia Italiana del Farmaco (Italy's health authority)

AITS: Adverse incident tracking system (medical devices sector)

ALT: Alanine aminotransferase (ALT = SGPT)

AM: Agence du Medicament (France)

AMA: American Medical Association

AMRH: African medicines regulatory harmonisation

ANADA: Abbreviated new animal drug application (US)

ANDA: Abbreviated new drug application

ANDS: Abbreviated new drug submission (Canada)

ANMV: Agence nationale du médicament vétérinaire (French vet medicines agency)

ANOVA: Analysis of Variance

ANZTPA: Australia and New Zealand therapeutic products agency (scheduled to come into force in 2016—replacing Australia's TGA and New Zealand's Medsafe)

AOAC: Association of official analytical chemists (US)

APEC: Asia-Pacific economic cooperation

APHIS: Animal and plant health inspection service (US)

APMA: Australian Pharmaceutical Manufacturers Association

APVMA: Australian pesticides and veterinary medicines authority (Australia)

AQL: Acceptable quality level

AR: Assessment report (EU)

ASAP: Accelerated Stability Assessment Program

ASCII: American standard code for information interchange quality assurance

ASDI: Acceptable single-dose intake

ASEAN: Association of Southeast Asian Nations

ASMF: Active substance master file

ASPR: Anonymised single patient report (formerly ASPP—anonymised single patient printout)

AST: Aspartate aminotransaminase (AST = SGOT)

B

BACPAC: Bulk active chemical post-approval changes (US)

BAN: British approved name

BAP: Biotechnology Action Programme

BARQA: British Association of Research Quality Assurance

BCS: Biopharmaceutics classification system

BDA: Bulgarian drug agency

BE: Bioequivalence

BGMA: British Generic Manufacturers Association

BIBRA: British Industrial Biological Research Association

BNF: British national formulary

BP: British Pharmacopoeia

BPC: British Pharmacopoeia Commission

BPC: Bulk pharmaceutical chemicals

BPCA: Best Pharmaceuticals in Children Act (US)

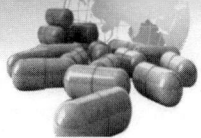

BRIC: Brazil, Russia, India and China
BRICK: Brazil, Russia, India, China and (South) Korea
BRICS: Brazil, Russia, India, China and South Africa
BROMI: Better regulation of over-the-counter medicines initiative

C

CADTH: Canadian agency for drugs and technologies in health (formerly CCOHTA)
CAMD: Competent authorities for medical devices
CAPRA: Canadian Association of Pharmaceutical Regulatory Affairs
CAS: Chemical abstract systems
CAT: Committee for advanced therapies (EMA)
CAVDRI: Collaboration agreement between veterinary drug registration institutions
CAVOMP: Clinical added value orphan medicinal product
CBER: Center for Biologics Evaluation and Research (US FDA)
CBG/MEB: Medicines Evaluation Board (the Netherlands)
CDC: Centers for Disease Control and Prevention (US)
CDEC: Canadian Drug Expert Committee (Canada)
CDER: Center for Drug Evaluation and Research (US FDA)
CDMA: Canadian Drug Manufacturers Association
CDR: Common Drug Review (Canada)
CDRH: Center for Devices and Radiological Health (US FDA)
CDSCO: Central Drug Standard Control Organization (India's clinical trials licensing authority)
CDSM: Committee on Dental and Surgical Materials (UK)
CE Mark: Conformité European (= approval for EU medical devices)
CEA: Cost-effectiveness analysis
CEC: Commission of the European Communities
CEE: Central and Eastern Europe
CEEC: Central and Eastern European Countries
CEFTA: Central Europe Free Trade Area
CEN: Comité Européan des Normes–European Committee for Standardization
CESP: Common European submissions platform
CFDA: China Food and Drug Administration (formerly State FDA–**SFDA**)
CFR: Code of Federal Regulations (US)
CFS: Certificate of free sale
CFSAN: Center for food safety and applied nutrition (US)
cGLP: Current good laboratory practice
cGMP: Current good manufacturing practice
CGP: Clinical Guidance Panel (Canada)

CH: Clinical hold

CHAI: Commission for Healthcare Audit and Inspection (UK)

CHMP: Committee for Medicinal Products for Human Use (EMA)

CHPA: Consumer Healthcare Products Association

CIA: Corporate Integrity Agreement (US)

CIOMS: Council for International Organizations of Medical Sciences (WHO)

CIRS: Centre for Innovation in Regulatory Science

CIS (countries): Commonwealth of Independent States (members are former Soviet Republic countries, currently including Armenia, Azerbaijan, Belarus, Kazakhstan, Kyrgyzstan, Moldova, Russia, Tajikistan, Usbekistan, Turkmenistan, Ukraine

CMA: Conditional marketing authorisation (US)

CMDh: Coordination Group for Mutual Recognition and Decentralised Procedures–Human (EMA)

CMDv: Coordination Group for Mutual Recognition and Decentralised Procedures–Veterinary (EMA)

CMS: Concerned member state (EU)

CMT: Convergent medical technologies

COA/CofA: Certificate of analysis

COE: Council of Europe

COMP: Committee for Orphan Medicinal Products (EMA)

COREPER: Committee of Permanent Representatives (i.e. Ambassadors) to the Community

COSHH: Control of Substances Hazardous to Health

COSTART: Coding symbols for a thesaurus of adverse reaction terms

CPAC: Central Pharmaceutical Affairs Council (Japan)

CPI: Critical path initiative (US)

CPMP: Committee for Proprietary Medicinal Products (EMA)

CSM: Committee on Safety of Medicines (UK)

CTD: Common technical document

CVM: Center for veterinary medicine (US)

CVMP: Committee for Medicinal Products for Veterinary Use (EMA)

CZ: Climatic zone

D

DAMOS: Drug application methodology with optical storage

DB: Device Bulletin (MHRA)

DCGI: India's regulatory authority (Directorate General of Health Services in the Ministry of Health and Family Welfare)

DCGI: Drugs Controller General of India

DCP: Decentralised procedure (EU)

DG: Directorate-General (at the European Commission)

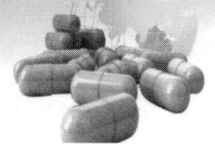

DGV: Direccao Geral de Veterinaria (Veterinary Medicines Agency) (Portugal)

DIA: Drug Information Association (US)

DIBD: Development international birth date

DMF: Drug master file

DMPK: Drug metabolism and pharmacokinetics

DMRC: Defective Medicines Report Centre (MHRA)

DMS: Document management system

DRA: Drug Regulatory Authority (non-EU)

DSRU: Drug Safety Research Unit (EMA)

DSUR: Development safety update report

E

EAI: Estimated acute intake

EC: European Commission

ECDC: European Centre for Disease Prevention and Control

EDMF: European drug master file

EDQM: European Directorate for the Quality of Medicines and Health Care

EEC: European Economic Community

ELA: Establishment license application (US)

EMA: European medicines agency (formerly European Medicines Evaluation Agency—EMEA)

EMEAA: Europe, Middle East Africa and Asia

EOQ: European Organization for Quality

EP/Ph Eur: European Pharmacopoeia

EPA: Environmental protection agency (US)

EPAA: European partnership for alternative approaches to animal testing

EPADES: European Parliament Document Exchange Server

EPAR: European public assessment report

EPC: European Pharmacopoeia Commission

EPHA: European public health alliance

EPITT: European pharmacovigilance issues tracking tool

ERA: European regulatory affairs

ESRA: European Society of Regulatory Affairs

ESTRI: Electronic Standards for the Transfer of Regulatory Information

ESVAC: European surveillance of veterinary antimicrobial consumption

EU: European Union

EU5: Group of countries comprising Germany, France, Italy, Spain and the UK

EUDRA: European Union Drug Regulatory Authorities

EUR-OP: EU Office for Publications

F

FDA: Food and Drug Administration (the US regulatory authority)

FDAAA: FDA Amendments Act

FDASIA: Food and Drug Administration Safety and Innovation Act

FR: Federal Register (US)

FrP: French Pharmacopoeia

FSIS: Food Safety and Inspection Service (US)

G

GATT: General Agreement on Tariffs and Trade

GCC (region): Gulf Cooperation Council (region)

GCC-DR: Gulf Central Committee for Drug Registration

GCG: Global Cooperation Group (ICH)

GCP: Good clinical practice

GCPv: Good clinical practice (veterinary)

GDP: Good distribution practice

GGP: Good guidance practice

GHTF: Global Harmonization Task Force

GLP: Good laboratory practice

GLPMA: Good Laboratory Practice Monitoring Authority (UK)

GMC: General Medical Council (UK)

GMiA: Generic Medicines Industry Association (Australia)

GMO: Genetically modified organism

GMP: Good manufacturing practice

GPIA: Generic Pharmaceutical Industry Association (US)

GPMSP: Good postmarketing surveillance practice (Japan)

GRB: Global Regulatory Board

GRP: Good regulatory practice

GVP: Good pharmacovigilance practice

GxP: General term for "good practice" quality guidelines and regulations, where "x" is the symbol for clinical, laboratory, manufacturing, pharmaceutical.

H

HCR: Holder of certificate of registration (South Africa)

HLT: High level term (in MedDRA)

HMA: Heads of Medicines Agencies (Human and Veterinary) (EU)

HMO: Health Maintenance Organization (US)

HMPC: Committee on herbal medicinal products (EMA)

HPB: Health Protection Board (Canada)

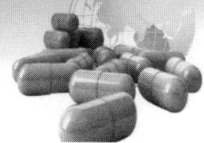

I

ICDRA: International Conference of Drug Regulatory Authorities

ICH: International Conference on Harmonisation (of Technical Requirements for Registration of Pharmaceuticals for Human use)

IMRDF: International Medical Device Regulatory Forum

INADA: Investigational new animal drug application

IND: Investigational new drug (US)

INDA: Investigational new drug application (US)

INDC: Investigational New Drug Committee

INN: International nonproprietary name

IP: Intellectual property

IUPAC: International Union of Pure and Applied Chemistry

J

JAN: Japanese Approved Name

JFDA: Jordan Food and Drug Administration

JIACRA: Joint Interagency Antimicrobial Consumption and Resistance Analysis

JNDA: Japanese New Drug Application

JP: Japanese Pharmacopoeia

JPMA: Japan Pharmaceutical Manufacturers Association

J-RMP: Japanese risk management plan (template)

M

MA: Marketing authorization

MAA: Marketing authorization application (EU)

MedDevs: Guidances outlining the requirements of the Medical Device Directive

MedDRA: Medical dictionary for regulatory activities

MEDEV: Medicine Evaluation Committee (EU)

MEDSAFE: New Zealand Medicines and Medical Devices Safety Authority

MENA: Middle East and North Africa

MHRA: Medicines and Healthcare products Regulatory Agency (UK's regulatory authority)

MHW: Ministry of Health and Welfare (Japan)

MIMS: Monthly Index of Medical Specialities (UK)

MINE: Medicines Information Network for Europe

MRFG: Mutual recognition facilitation group (EMA)

N

NDA: New drug application (US)

NDAC: New Drug Advisory Committee (India)

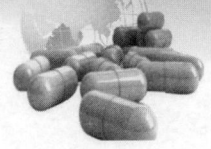

NDMA: Non-prescription Drug Manufacturers Association (US)

NDS: New drug submission (Canada)

NF: National Formulary

NICHD: National Institute of Child Health and Human Development (US)

NIH: National Institutes of Health (US)

NIHR: National Institute for Health Research (UK)

NPCB: National Pharmaceutical Control Bureau (Malaysia)

O

OD: Orphan drug

ODA: Orphan Drugs Act (US)

ODD: Orphan drug designation

OMP: Orphan medicinal product

OOPD: Office of orphan products development (US FDA)

OPA: Office of public affairs (US)

OPD: Original pack dispensing

OPE: Office of planning and evaluation (US)

ORA: Office of regulatory affairs (US FDA)

P

PA: Product authorisation

PAL: Pharmaceutical Affairs Law (Japan)

PAR: Preliminary assessment report

PAS: Public affairs specialist (US)

PASS: Post-authorisation safety study

PBAC: Pharmaceutical Benefits Advisory Committee (Australia)

PBS: Pharmaceutical benefit scheme (Australia)

PCG: Product coordination group (EU)

PCT: Primary care trust (UK)

PDG: Pharmacopoeial discussion group

PDMA: Prescription Drug Marketing Act (US)

PDP: Product development protocols (for medical devices) (US)

PDUFA: Prescription Drug User Fee Act (US)

PE: Pharmacoeconomics

PEAG: Pharmacovigilance expert advisory group (MHRA)

PECA: Protocol to the Europe agreement on conformity assessment and acceptance of industrial products

PEFRAS: Pan European Federation of Regulatory Affairs

PEI: Paul-Ehrlich-Institut [Federal Institute for Vaccines and Biomedicines (one of the two German regulatory agencies)]

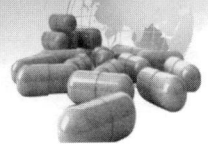

Ph Eur: European Pharmacopoeia

PHARMO: Institute for Drug Outcomes Research (the Netherlands)

PhPID: Pharmaceutical product identifiers (EU)

PhRMA: Pharmaceutical Research and Manufacturers of America

PHS: Public health service (US)

PIIGS: Portugal, Ireland, Italy, Greece and Spain

PL: Product license (US)

PMDA: Japan's regulatory agency—the Pharmaceutical and Medical Devices Agency (within the Ministry of Health, Labor and Welfare—**MHLW**)

PMF: Plant master file (US and Canada)

PMPRB: Patented Medicines Prices Review Board (Canada)

PMS study: Post-marketing safety study

PPRS: Pharmaceutical price regulation scheme

PPSR: Proposed Paediatric Study Request (US)

PR: Pulse rate

Q

QA: Quality assurance

QALY: Quality-adjusted life year

QbD: Quality by design

QC: Quality control

QSIT: Quality Systems Inspection Technique (US FDA)

QTPP: Quality target product profile

QUAMED: Quality Medicines for All

QWP: Quality Working Party (EMA)

R

R&D: Research and development

RAMA: Remote access for marketing authorizations (MHRA)

RAPS: Regulatory Affairs Professionals Society (US)

RHSC: Regulatory Harmonization Steering Committee

RI: Regulatory intelligence

S

SBA/SBOA: Summary basis of approval (US)

SFDA: Saudi Food and Drug Authority

SmPAR: Summary Pharmacovigilance Assessment Report (EU)

T

TAG: Therapeutic Advisory Group

TGA: Therapeutic goods administration

THMPD: Traditional herbal medicinal products directive

THMRS: Traditional herbal medicines registration scheme

THR: Traditional herbal registration

TOPRA: The Organization for Professionals in Regulatory Affairs

TSA: Therapeutic Substances Act

U

USP: United States Pharmacopoeia

USP-DI: United States Pharmacopeia-Drug Information

USP-NF: United States Pharmacopeia-National Formulary

V

VDD: Veterinary Drugs Directorate (Canada)

VF: Ventricular failure

VHP: Voluntary harmonization procedure

VNeeS: Veterinary non-eCTD electronic submission

VPC: Veterinary Products Committee (UK)

W

WHO: World Health Organization

WRAC: Worldwide Regulatory Affairs Committee

WTO: World Trade Organization

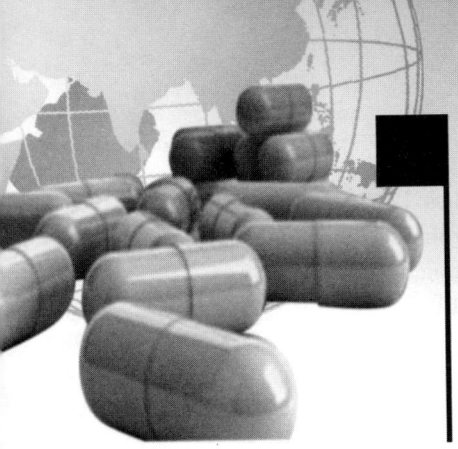

Index